Crip
Kinship

Crip Kinship

The Disability Justice
& Art Activism
of Sins Invalid

SHAYDA KAFAI

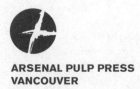

ARSENAL PULP PRESS
VANCOUVER

CRIP KINSHIP
Copyright © 2021 by Shayda Kafai

THIRD PRINTING: 2023

ARSENAL PULP PRESS
Suite 202 – 211 East Georgia St.
Vancouver, BC V6A 1Z6
Canada
arsenalpulp.com

Arsenal Pulp Press acknowledges the xʷməθkʷəy̓əm (Musqueam), Sḵwx̱wú7mesh
(Squamish), and səl̓ilwətaʔɬ (Tsleil-Waututh) Nations, custodians of the traditional,
ancestral, and unceded territories where our office is located. We pay respect to their
histories, traditions, and continuous living cultures and commit to accountability,
respectful relations, and friendship.

Cover and interior design by Jazmin Welch
Cover art by Kah Yangni
Copy edited by Doretta Lau
Proofread by Catharine Chen

Printed and bound in Canada

Library and Archives Canada Cataloguing in Publication:
Title: Crip kinship : the disability justice & art activism of Sins Invalid / Shayda Kafai.
Names: Kafai, Shayda, author.
Identifiers: Canadiana (print) 20210212411 | Canadiana (ebook) 20210212500 |
    ISBN 9781551528649 (softcover) | ISBN 9781551528656 (HTML)
Subjects: LCSH: Sins Invalid (Organization) | LCSH: Artists with disabilities—
    California—San Francisco. | LCSH: Artists with disabilities—Political activity—
    California—San Francisco. | LCSH: Political art—California—San Francisco
Classification: LCC N8355 .K34 2021 | DDC 704/.087—dc23

To our disabled, queer of color doulas and ancestors.

To Amy for leading me home.

Contents

FOREWORD

I was fortunate to grow up in the San Francisco Bay Area at a time when there was a lot of emerging radical art there. As a young, queer radical with a hope for sex around every corner, I gravitated toward the many underground art scenes, queer cultural spaces, and illicit drugs spots that were available and accessible to me in the early 1980s.

Despite going year after year to queer film festivals and late-night meetings for "Third World" peoples (shout out to Mandela Arts!), I never, *ever* found a space where brown, disabled, politically sharp, and snarky queers were centered or even represented. It was a nexus of identities, politics, and aesthetics that didn't exist.

In 2005, when Leroy Moore, Amanda Coslor, Todd Herman, and I started discussing the project that became Sins Invalid, it was going to be a one-time performance. I knew that disabled people of color needed to see ourselves mirrored. I knew that *I* needed to see myself—my own gender non-conforming crip body—reflected back to me. What I didn't realize was how much I and other people needed to see the multiplicity of our non-normative, non-able bodyminds ... until that first, then second, then third show happened.

Back in 2005 I did not imagine the future that we would create together. It amazes me that we now have third-generation disability justice folks. I remember the first time I met somebody from the disability community who didn't come from a Disability Rights framework, but from Disability Justice. And I remember being humbled and amazed and tickled and delighted to realize that there were people who were coming up in this framework.

I did not expect Sins Invalid (Sins, to those close to us) to blossom the way it did, because I didn't fully grasp how novel one of Sins' central messages was for so many people. I'd thought it a given that every human is beautiful and powerful; I thought this was more than evident! It shouldn't be such a far-out concept that all humans are valuable and that the world should be organized around our collective and individual value. And that means including people with disabilities, including Black, brown, Indigenous, queer, gender non-conforming, and trans crips.

Please don't get it twisted—my childhood was far from picture perfect. I also have a sharp critique of capitalism's ongoing reduction of life to simple components of an economic equation in which a disabled body is rendered useless. But in the hours and years of healing work that I struggled through, I clung tightly to the spiritual tenet that all beings are sacred, which, after years, I finally internalized to include me.

When I think about the current moment, it appears that ableism is doing better than ever. As capitalism continues to define work, ableism becomes more and more entrenched in every generation. During the pandemic, eugenic practices increased and no alarms were sounded. Down the street from where I live, hospitals were denying disabled people access to ventilators so that non-disabled people could have them.

And at the same time, the pandemic has set the stage for us to experience a mass disabling.

Many people have been given the opportunity to look at their work and question whether it's worth risking their lives, particularly at a J.O.B. that exploits them and extracts from them. Of course, within cis-heteropatriarchal capitalism, others were forced to work. As people with disabilities, we have always had to ask ourselves, is this job worth the labor we have to put into it?

Crip life invites us into fierce creativity. Because the world continues to treat us as worthless, creating new worlds is a matter of survival for us. Dreaming is a matter of survival. This is part of the power of Sins; we dream new crip worlds together. We dream without shame. We dream out loud and in public.

I've always had a relationship with all the living world, including minerals and rocks. Growing up near the ocean, across the street from Golden Gate Park, meant waking up to the smell of salt in the air, the sounds of sea lions barking, and touching plants and pine trees every day. Now, at fifty-four (that's at least seventy in crip years) I find myself deeply connected again to the non-human universe, inspired by the beauty of all that is not human.

I used to have expectations for humans that I don't anymore. It's sobering to experience a pandemic and see how difficult change is for people. It's sobering to see how much pain the ocean can be in and how few fucks humans can give. It's painfully sobering. I've had to do some serious expectation management of our species. You can only get heartbroken so many times before you recognize the nature of the beast.

But like all things, this beast is not all good or all bad. I deeply love my partner and my community of friends and am myself deeply loved.

I've been broken in relationships, and I've been saved in relationships. Sins Invalid reflects my learnings up until now, and I'm grateful to Shayda Kafai for being in community and in integrity while creating this book. I'm grateful to each reader who wants to explore the universe of Sins Invalid.

In gratitude,

Patty Berne, Berkeley, California
supported by Cory Silverberg, Toronto, 2021

INTRODUCTION

"You are not too sick, too disabled, too sad, too crazy, too ugly, too fat, or too weird. We live in a white supremacist, patriarchal, ableist culture that values oppressive standards for the sake of centralizing power and making profit. Our ostracism is a result of this system that demonizes difference and not a reflection of your worth, value, ability to be loved, etc. You are not the problem. You are perfect."
—ACCESS CENTERED MOVEMENT

This book is a love letter, an abundant offering written out of need. Need communicates, says disabled communities have wisdom, says we survive true when we declare and cocreate a world that honors us, a world where we are never too much. Need says persistence, says crip[1] magic, says now. I lean into this exploration of need for all of us, but especially for the disabled, crip, chronically ill, Mad[2] community who are *also*: *also* queer, gender nonconforming, or transgender; *also* people of color; *also* the incarcerated many, the immigrant many. All of us, *also*.

I have written this book because my own disabled, Mad, queer, femme of color bodymind[3] needs to remember that ours is a legacy of resistance and revolution. Even as we live in a systemic, oppressive network of ableism, sanism, audism,[4] racism, cis-heteropatriarchy, classism, and capitalism, we gather and manifest liberatory practices—we always have. Our disabled, queer of color bodyminds[5] confront erasure and alienation. We actively revise the reductive narrative that we are inherently too damaged or too broken, that we are undeserving of celebration, joy, and beauty. For those of us who have been told otherwise, or who might never have had access to our crip, queer stories, Sins Invalid exists as a tether rooting us back to ourselves. Since their creation in 2006, the San Francisco Bay Area–based performance project provides the community Disability Justice–informed evenings of multidisciplinary art, workshops, and educational trainings that center the knowledges of disabled, queer, gender nonconforming, and transgender artist-activists of color. *Crip Kinship: The Disability Justice & Art Activism of Sins Invalid* explores their work and demonstrates how all our bodyminds, communities, and movements can benefit from Sins Invalid's resilient disabled, queer of color future-making.

As I sit at my desk thinking about community, I pull a card from Cristy C. Road's *Next World Tarot* deck. Cristy is a Cuban American queer femme, punk singer, and artist-activist. Her art and her words render intersectionality medicinal. In the booklet she has written to accompany the deck, she asks us: "How do we hold each other up in a world where oppression can be louder than self-love? … The Next World Tarot is a femme hacker, eager to out the truth and tired of compromising her mind and body for stability." This deck is social justice activism, social justice art, and accordingly, the card I pull to guide the writing of this introduction, the king of cups, is not depicted as a white man on a throne. For Cristy, the king of cups is a brown femme with long flowing hair. The king of cups sits on her wheelchair, wearing comfortable, loose-fitting purple pants, an olive T-shirt, and a peacock feather tucked behind her ear. This femme is barefoot and her wheelchair rolls on a growing, living path. With a serene face, she offers us a lotus flower in her palms. Cristy's king of cups is crip, queer, decolonial radiance. She brings with her "awareness of logic while maintaining a soft open heart"; with her call for balance, she invites us to harness our "collected rage and unconditional love."[6]

Crip Kinship manifests a present moment of "collected rage and unconditional love" for all our bodyminds. Led by the generational and communal knowledges of disabled, queer of color communities, in this present moment all our collective needs are met, regardless of how frequently ableism, racism, cis-heteropatriarchy, and all the systems of oppression tell us to wait, tell us later, or tell us never.[7] Dear reader, this moment is not solely aspirational. Sins Invalid reminds us that it is happening in our communities now in slow, messy, poignant, and nuanced ways. It is happening because the most marginalized of us have together willed it, given time to it, and fed it with "collected rage and unconditional love." This movement is called Disability Justice and it is the liberatory framework Sins Invalid uses to move us closer toward our collective liberation. I offer Sins Invalid and their strategies for living and thriving in this world as medicine for a contemporary moment that is precarious and that has left us exhausted and experiencing an unrivaled instability.

I began this book project earnestly and slowly, in crip time,[8] in the summer of 2016. I began in response to a need for survival stories, a need for hope stories. I needed to experience generative strategies for our collective perseverance despite all of the loss. That summer, I had read two news stories in particular about disabled folks which refused to leave me. One took place outside of Tokyo, Japan, and the other in Appleton, Wisconsin. Although I talk about these two moments in great detail in chapter 5, "Artmaking as Evidence," what I will say here is that these were stories of crip death and crip loss that left me enraged and overwhelmed. It was 2016 and nondisabled supremacy and eugenics had raised the stakes again, continuing to render our disabled lives disposable, again.

In need of community and the hoping-making that is Sins Invalid, I returned to my dissertation. I had written about the performance project and their art-activism, but in many ways, I had removed my voice and the poetry of it all. After finishing graduate school in 2014, I knew that I needed to let the work rest so that I could grow something entirely different from the composted collection of what it was. That summer, I explored, conducted more interviews, and began writing. I began writing to locate myself and to find disabled, queer of color kinship in all our resistance and determination, in all the lessons we, in our cultural moment, desperately needed.

———————

As I complete this introduction now in the year 2020, sitting at my desk in Pomona, California, the list to describe our collective present in the United States leaves me similarly enraged and overwhelmed. Fires in California damaged land, properties, and took lives; the country struggled to breathe; states experienced extreme weather, including record-breaking heat, fires, and hurricanes. Right now, we are surrounded by the tangible effects of the COVID-19 pandemic as positive cases in the US, particularly Los Angeles, surge; Black men, Black women, and Black trans women continue to be murdered; millions of people marched in protests organized by Black Lives Matter this summer, resulting in one of the largest social justice movements in our history[9]—and this is not just a list of facts. Each of these issues has resonance and is deeply felt in our bodyminds and in our spirits.

We have never needed Sins Invalid's Disability Justice practice for collective liberation and collective access with as much urgency as we do now, whether we are disabled or not. Those of us who are most privileged need to humble ourselves now and learn from those who are most marginalized, from those who have struggled through and who refuse erasure. Abolitionist community lawyer and organizer Talila A. Lewis writes that the gift of the most marginalized is their "dream work": "Indeed, dreaming is among the most difficult and brave kinds of advocacy work ... When we create space for ourselves and others to dream, we embody recurring hope, active love, critical resistance, and radical change. We are reminded that those who came before us dreamed of that which no one thought could exist—that their dreams are the reasons that we now are living the 'impossible.'"[10]

Perhaps the most compelling survival tool that disabled, queer, gender nonconforming, and transgender communities of color have is their dreamwork. Dreaming is not passive. In dreaming, our communities materialize a world where, through fury and love, transformation in all its rebelliousness thrives.

Sins Invalid's artist-activists nourish and produce distinctly from this place. With their crip wisdom and Disability Justice practice, the performance project becomes a resistance manual, a guidebook for how to survive resiliently without compromising our intersecting identities and without sacrificing our bodyminds. They call this place a "crip-centric liberated zone,"[11] a place where, through art, activism, community workshops, and trainings we can enter into a present where all our bodyminds are valid, beautiful, and revolutionary, a present where we can live liberated from oppression. Within a crip-centric liberated zone, we can reimagine what insistent and courageous disabled, queer of color living can truly do.

———————

Dear reader, Sins Invalid's dreamwork and art-activism is not just for the disabled, queer of color many. It is for all of us, for all spaces and peoples in need of nourishment and thriving in our ableist, racist, and cis-heteropatriarchal world. The performance project reveals that art made by an intersectional Disability Justice community holds power; it holds the potential to motivate us to question what we have been taught about our bodyminds, about who we have been taught is perpetually disempowered, and about who does and does not have a voice.

This is what *Crip Kinship* offers: a mapping of intersecting crip networks, of thriving structures of crip love gathered and shared. This is a book of collective witnessing, a gridwork of fibers, a persistent and complex arrangement of all things tender and kindred. It is about an opening into a defiant present, a welcoming into a place, liberated.

———————

Remembering the Erased

To begin this journey, we must first remember the forgotten. So many disabled queer and disabled of color communities raised fists in solidarity during the mainstream Disability Rights Movement.[12] They protested during sit-ins, rolled, limped, crawled, and walked in marches, and envisioned loving, accessible crip futures. Truth: I wouldn't have had the access, pride, and political empowerment I have today as a disabled, Mad, queer, femme of color were it not for the labor and cultural shifts of these activists and dreamers. There were, however, also communal erasures within the mainstream Disability Rights Movement. The movement, including its historical retellings, primarily centered the organizing of white disabled activists; the academic extension of the movement, Disability Studies, similarly centered the experiences of white scholars.[13]

To begin the process of remembering, I call on the labor, organizing, and crip wisdom of disabled activists of color Vilissa Thompson and Alice Wong. Vilissa is a Black disabled activist, social worker, and founder of the website *Ramp Your Voice!* She writes, "[Disabled activists of color] have ALWAYS been here since the beginning of the movement, but if you were to go by the history books that discusses disability rights, you will not see our faces, voices, or stories shared freely."[14] Vilissa appeals for communal acknowledgement and recognition, rather than exclusion. Her annual project of featuring Black disabled community leaders during Black History Month is part of her dedication to affirming a history of disabled leadership and advocacy that we need to remember and archive. Her website was one of the first places I learned about the works and erasures of Johnnie Lacy, Don Galloway, Bradley Lomax, and Joyce Jackson.

Alice Wong similarly holds space for the lived experiences and activisms of the diverse disability community of which so many of us are a part. As a Disability Justice activist, writer, media maker, and founder of the Disability Visibility Project, she writes about having felt "like a unicorn" in mainstream disability activist circles: "As a disabled Asian American woman, I am not a unicorn by any stretch. And yet, there are times in my activism when I rarely see people like myself."[15] This longing for community and intersectional recognition is not new. It is something that many mainstream activist movements have struggled through.[16] At the heart of it is the desire to acknowledge the labor of people of color[17] and the queer and transgender communities who were also disabled and who also dreamt disabled dreams of change. In partnership with StoryCorps, Alice pushes back against the mainstream Disability Rights Movement's tendency toward erasure by recording and preserving the oral narratives of disabled community members who are queer and who are of color for the Library of Congress.

Alice and Vilissa are among an expansive, fierce network of disabled activists who are reminding us of our disabled, queer of color kin and contemporaries. It is celebratory to return to this forgotten lineage and to highlight the folks dreaming our crip futures. It is a reminder of how truly revolutionary recognition can be.

———————

The call to acknowledge disabled, queer of color activists, cultural workers, and scholars confirms the reality that so many of us have always known: ableism always intersects with other systems of oppression. For a movement to truly embrace the diverse disabled many, it also needs to recognize the reality that many of us are *also*. The mainstream Disability

Rights Movement's focus on whiteness, maleness, and heteronorma-
tivity simply does not hold space for all our bodyminds.[18] I call on the
intervention and words of Black, lesbian, feminist ancestor Audre Lorde
here and her writings about having breast cancer and about how her
body's experiences were always mediated through a medical gaze that
was at once patriarchal and racialized. I think of her urging that "There
is no such thing as a single-issue struggle because we do not live single-
issue lives."[19] Our stories and our histories must accurately reflect the
complexity of our lives. If we do not do this, then we are complicit in
leaving so many of us behind.

Patricia (Patty) Berne (she/they), the cofounder and the executive
and artistic director of Sins Invalid, notes that an alarming pitfall of
the mainstream Disability Rights Movement is its singular focus on
disability as its primary identity. As one of the collective founders of
Disability Justice, Patty writes:

> The histories of white supremacy and ableism are inextricably entwined,
> created in the context of colonial conquest and capitalist domination.
> One cannot look at the history of US slavery, the stealing of Indigenous
> lands, and US imperialism without seeing the way that white supremacy
> uses ableism to create a lesser/ 'other' group of people that is deemed
> less worthy/abled/smart/capable. A single-issue civil rights framework
> is not enough to explain the full extent of ableism and how it operates in
> society. We can only truly understand ableism by tracing its connections
> to heteropatriarchy, white supremacy, colonialism, and capitalism.[20]

To create change-making that is radical, lasting, and truly liberatory,
we need to integrate intersectionality into our movement building
work. We, as Vilissa reminds us, have always been here, our disabled

bodyminds aware of the long history of eugenics, scientific racism, colonialism, and capitalist productivity that labels us disposable.[21] We, in all our crip communal glory, are too valuable to be synthesized into one identity. We require a dynamic homeplace of absolute witnessing.

The Roots of Disability Justice

Beginning in 2006, Sins Invalid grew out of the gaps of the mainstream Disability Rights Movement, out of its lack, and out of a desire to create what bell hooks calls "a community of resistance,"[22] a place where we as disabled queer of color community are seen as our unapologetically beautiful whole selves. This community of resistance grounds itself in affirmation, crip love, and remembrance.

Before learning Sins Invalid's origin story, it is important for us to first understand Disability Justice, the "movement building framework"[23] that grounds the performance project's art-activism. Since Sins Invalid began a year after Disability Justice was established, many of their core community of cultural workers and artmakers were involved in crafting Disability Justice as a framework. In 2005, disabled, queer of color activists Patty Berne, Mia Mingus, and Stacey Milbern conceived Disability Justice in community with Leroy F. Moore Jr.—the cofounder of Sins Invalid and the founder of Krip-Hop Nation—and disabled, trans activists Sebastian Margaret and Eli Clare. As a movement building framework, Disability Justice not only responds to the gaps in the mainstream Disability Rights Movement, but also offers principles framed in wholeness and persistence. Serving as the second wave of the Disability

Rights Movement, Disability Justice begins to formulate strategies of survival for all our disabled, queer of color bodyminds.

———————

In 2015, Patty began to notice that people were using Disability Justice outside of its disabled, queer of color origins. Ten years after its initial collective birthing, it was being misinterpreted. A simple Google search of "disability justice" revealed that the phrase had become synonymous with legal aid and online support for the disability community. Disability Justice community activists had also observed people adding "justice" to the word disability without actually enacting any Disability Justice politics or practices.[24] Perhaps most troubling, Patty also noticed that the framework was being misused and co-opted primarily by white academics and activists who were using Disability Justice as a framework, while the community who created it, the communities that it was meant to sustain and support, had not had a chance to define its parameters.[25] These occurrences pushed Patty, Sins Invalid's artist-activists, and fellow disabled, queer and trans of color communities to establish a written record and a cohesive definition of Disability Justice.

What resulted was a 2015 blog post on Sins Invalid's website entitled "Disability Justice—A Working Draft by Patty Berne." This collaboratively written working draft included a brief history of Disability Justice, along with its ten working principles. A year after this blog post, the Sins Invalid artist-activist community completed and published the first comprehensive Disability Justice text. Entitled *Skin, Tooth, and Bone— The Basis of Movement is Our People: A Disability Justice Primer*, it not only introduced Disability Justice and expanded the originally drafted principles, but also provided strategies for implementing Disability Justice and its principles to community organizers unfamiliar with ableism. The primer's second edition was released in 2019 after Sins Invalid solicited and applied community feedback. It includes new sections that discuss audism and Deafness[26] and the intersection of ableism and our current climate crisis.

Perhaps most importantly, the primer ends with timelines of Sins Invalid and of Disability Justice. Serving as an archive of memory and reclamation, the Disability Justice timeline does not begin in 2005, but with Harriet Tubman in 1820. It includes Frida Kahlo, Audre Lorde, Cherrie Moraga, and Gloria Anzaldúa. This timeline excavates a history of activists, artists, and writers who were practicing Disability Justice before it was a named concept. It also serves as a collection of inter-sectional crip memory, calling forward people we may not have known were disabled. It is an active reminder that we must remember and acknowledge who in our communities has been doing this work.

This cripped, queered, and decolonial timeline ensures that once you arrive to the end of the primer, there is no mistaking what Disability Justice is or who created it. There is no misinterpreting that Disability Justice came into being when disabled, queer people of color gathered in conversation, exhausted and ready to weave a collective, empowering praxis of love and resistance, together. In a world that has delegitimized the wisdom, beauty, and resilience of crip living and crip ancestry, Disability Justice answers a gut desire for authentic and communal recognition outside the frame-works of ableism, racism, and cis-heteropatriarchy. Sins Invalid flourished from this same place of desire, fatigue, and persistence and hosted their first performance a year after Disability Justice began.

Writing Ourselves (Myself) In

In writing this book, I have thought a lot about what can happen when we tell our own bodymind stories, when we resist erasure and write ourselves *in*. How can telling our bodymind stories instigate change? How do we alter our timelines and collaboratively create new futures when we learn our histories and share our bodymind stories? How does our relationship to ourselves change when we proclaim our bodyminds in all our rolling, limping, drooling, frenetically stimming, and Mad glory? In her book *Living a Feminist Life*, writer and scholar Sara Ahmed discusses willfulness. She writes that when feminists, women of color, colonized peoples, and people from different classes protest and insist on naming themselves, they are often viewed as willful.[27] Sins Invalid re-empowers our disabled, queer of color selves so that we can reclaim our willful resistance as a bold tool. They invite us to construct and revel in a liberatory place, to recover from ableist, racist, cis-heteropatriarchal elimination, and to write ourselves *in* despite being told that we do not matter. Willfully writing ourselves *in* in this way becomes the responsibility of our artists, writers, and activists; it becomes the responsibility of all of us who dream. Sins Invalid carries our communities forward by teaching us how to cocreate a future where our communities can thrive as the crip, queer of color bodyminds we are.

I follow Sins Invalid's call for willfulness in writing this book. It is with politicized intention that I write myself in by using first person *I* and first-person plural *we* throughout the book or by turning outward and speaking directly to *you*. It is a willful act to name myself as a disabled, Mad, queer femme of color in a society that tells me to hide my Madness and queerness, that tells me to avoid claiming my identities with pride. This urging comes from Critical Disability Studies scholars and activists who argue that it is a political act to name ourselves as disabled, and who say that language and the words we choose matter.

—————

The artists, activists, scholars, and educators that I have chosen to be in conversation with throughout this book are another way of writing myself *in*. I offer the following pages as a tender, focused place with disabled, queer of color citations of community who are, for me, in dialogue with Sins Invalid. I return to Sara Ahmed, as she informs my thinking about what it means to cite and to gather citations. She argues that citations are not passive things we include into our writings; they chronicle specific histories and are a political practice: "Citation is how we acknowledge our debt to those who came before; those who helped us find our way."[28] The citations in this book create pathways of disabled, queer of color knowledge production. For me, they serve as a personal practice of uplifting community, giving shout-outs, and offering the knowledge magic of resistance writers and activists whose words arouse change.

My hope is that these citations will become sparks, launching points that can send you on your own search, building your own living, breathing citational archive of artist-activists. We, dear reader, come from somewhere. We move through this world supported by determined and affirming bodyminds, and though the connections might not always be legible, we are always in community. Citations remind us of this, and maybe that is also what citations are: they are the phrases that bolster us and give us electric, stimmy joy. How will you resist bodymind elimination? How will you write yourself *in*?

—————

Lastly, a Practice of Care

As you make your way through this book, you might find that your own unique identities and life journeys place you squarely in conversation with Sins Invalid and their work. Perhaps this is the first time you are reading a book that reimagines the future making and art-activism of disabled, queer of color communities. Maybe you are learning the word "ableism" for the first time. Returning to the idea of this book as a love letter and an offering, wherever you are located, know that you are welcome.

———————

In the practice of disabled, queer of color love and resilience, I ask you to read this book with care. Care might mean reading in slowness with frequent breaks. It might mean pausing to journal or to gather the citations that are lifegiving or the lessons from Sins Invalid that you plan to apply to your own communal or daily practice. Care might also refer to honoring your tangible bodymind needs: closing your eyes, stretching, breaking to eat, or acknowledging the rise of feelings and pausing to cry. Move and process as you need to, dear reader. May it launch you toward cultivating the soil and the seedlings of your own liberatory future.

CHAPTER I

Sins Invalid's Origin Story

Sins Invalid began in 2006 over crip love, food, and conversation among Bay Area disability activists and friends Patty Berne (she/they) and Leroy F. Moore Jr. (he/him); Patty is a Japanese-Haitian, disabled, queer, gender nonbinary artist-activist and Leroy is an African American, krip[29] poet, community historian, and artist-activist. As they sat in La Peña, a cultural center created by Chilean exiles on the edge of Berkeley and Oakland, Patty remembers that, "Like many good stories, the early threads of this one were woven over dinner, a large bowl of saffron-laced *paella* steaming on the table between two good friends."[30] That day, they began by talking about Leroy's artistic collaboration with filmmaker and photographer Todd Herman. Leroy had just completed *Forbidden Acts*, a twelve-minute piece that centered his sexuality and his poetry.

When Patty and Leroy spoke about crip sexuality, they spoke aware of their crip fierceness and lust; they began with the awareness that for so long, their crip beauty and sexuality had been juxtaposed against the deeply felt ableist beliefs that they are "less than, undesirable, and pitiable"[31] simply because they are disabled. Their bodyminds had felt the

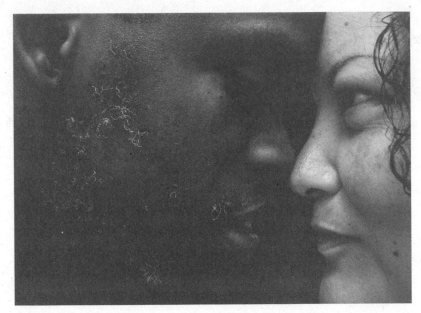

Leroy Moore and Patty Berne. Photo by Amal Kouttab, courtesy of Sins Invalid.

historical impacts of eugenics, forced sterilizations, and ugly laws;[32] they felt the ableist assumption that as disabled folks, they must be childlike and desexual. Patty remembers telling Leroy, "'We should have a venue for this, where we would not just be the token Other. Where would that be?' And we thought, 'Oh, our own venue!'"[33] Sins Invalid's beginnings grew here among saffron, among their sexy bodyminds craving recognition. That evening at La Peña was the first spark, that cutting flash of bright light that initiated the performance project into action.

————————

It Begins with Intersectionality

Early on in their journey, Patty and Leroy connected with Todd Herman and fellow artist Amanda Coslor, and soon, the group of four nurtured Sins Invalid into being. Patty writes that Todd and Amanda "offered to collaborate, contributing massively toward the aesthetics, contacts, and available resources. Sins Invalid then had a dedicated core group, more-over, a family."[34] Specifically, Todd and Amanda brought with them a grant that they had yet to fulfill from Theatre Bay Area, a nonprofit arts organization. Serendipitously, they had received the grant for the specific purpose of putting together a show about the intersections of disability and sexuality. This was a moment of true alchemy.

The artist-activists arrived together with the communal understanding that a disabled, queer of color art space needed to exist, one that was mindful of Disability Justice, one where conversations surrounding disability could occur in unison with conversations about sexuality, beauty, autonomy, and desire. The disability community was in need of a cultural shift, an acknowledgement of the crip beauty and sexuality that Patty and Leroy knew to be true. Our community needed a place of intersectional bodymind appreciation and space holding.

Intersectionality as a framework considers the layered ways our identities converge, engage, and inform one another. Originating with the work of lawyer and critical race scholar Kimberlé Crenshaw, and serving as the first principle of Disability Justice, Sins Invalid defines intersectionality this way: "Simply put, this principle says that we are many things, and they all impact us. We are not only disabled, we are also each coming from a specific experience of race, class, sexuality, age, religious background, geographic location, immigration status, and more. Depending on context, we all have areas where we experience privilege, as well as areas of oppression ... We gratefully embrace the nuance that this principle brings to our lived experiences, and the ways it shapes the perspectives we offer."[35]

Sins Invalid cannot practice Disability Justice or progress as a performance project without acknowledging the intersections of our bodyminds. It is a framework that fills in the gaps of the mainstream Disability Rights Movement and creates new imaginings of what can happen when we acknowledge our unique bodymind experiences.

More than a lens, intersectionality also results in relentless and unshamed embraces of our disabled, queer of color bodyminds. Sins Invalid practices intersectionality in their work and they invite us to participate in a similar pursuit. The fact that we are made up of many things becomes an opening, an invocation that we deserve to move purposefully through this world as our full and intricate selves. I turn to Cara Page's monologue during Sins Invalid's 2008 performance to provide us with a clear description of what it means to *enact* intersectionality. Standing on stage at San Francisco's Brava Theater, Cara, a Black feminist queer cultural memory worker, addresses the audience: "Sins Invalid asks of you unapologetically to love all of your parts, your disabled parts, queer parts, radical parts, erotic parts, political parts, without exception, without judgment, without normality or pathology, without sacrifice ... welcome the possibilities that you are whole and perfect, that we are whole and perfect."

Cara's monologue presents us with what intersectionality yields and elicits: we all are welcomed into a liberated place where we can confirm and honor the myriad parts of ourselves. For Sins Invalid, this practice becomes foundational to what they create and how they celebrate disabled, queer of color bodyminds. With their art-activism, they encourage us to view ourselves without shame, in wholeness and in affirmation.

―――――――

Initially, Patty and Leroy envisioned Sins Invalid as a small-scale, single-evening event for close friends at a local café. When the call for artists was released, Patty remembers that they were overwhelmed with interest. The desire for homecoming could not have been communicated more clearly; Patty and Leroy were not the only ones who desired disabled, queer of color representation, visibility, and magic. The community was collectively exhausted and frustrated by the mainstream Disability Rights Movement's erasure of disabled folks who were queer, gender nonconforming, transgender, and of color; it was an exhaustion of the spirit. The artist-activist space that Sins Invalid created became an opening palm, a gesture of welcoming, a statement: *we have always been here, too*. After their first night of multidisciplinary performance art, the disabled, queer of color community desired for more whole, beautiful, and radically liberated representations of themselves, and so, Sins Invalid grew.

―――――――

By 2008, two years after what was meant to be a one-time performance, Sins Invalid officially became a performance project grown out of need and in solidarity with crip family and love. They used the initial funding from Theatre Bay Area to support their work for their first four years.[36] Patty shared that, as is common in the early months of any organization, the group of four also had to use their own personal money and in-kind services to bolster and breathe life into the performance project. The studio space behind Patty and visual artist Micah Bazant's home in Berkeley, California, was renamed Sins Central and became Sins Invalid's central hub, a place where its members and supporters would meet to organize, plan, and reimagine what disabled, queer of color living could look like.

Since 2008, Sins Invalid has created a new home where disabled, queer of color artist-activists can teach their lessons of survival and thriving, a place where community can "see"—in all the diverse, accessible ways we "see"— sexuality and beauty no longer judged based on their proximity to whiteness, cis-heteropatriarchy, and nondisability. Patty and Leroy's Disability Justice–informed content fostered inclusivity, whole bodymind liberation, and radical crip visibility as healing for the communities that the mainstream Disability Rights Movement had left behind.

The broadening and politicization of beauty and sexuality continues to be a critical intervention for the performance project. It is profound for us to learn how to reframe beauty and sexuality as actions and as crip bodymind manifestations of radiance, especially when we are told that sexuality and beauty are unattainable impossibilities for us. Patty, Leroy, Todd, and Amanda[37] initiated Sins Invalid as a living, growing repository of performances, histories, stories, and workshops that remind us that crip beauty is tongue-slurring. It is dance-swaying with canes and in wheelchairs. It is glittery stimmy-ness. It is neurodiverse and Mad minds manic-dreaming. Crip beauty happens when we embrace our bodyminds as the lustrous, intersectional sources of energy that they are.

———————

Imagination First

Creating new realities requires imagination. It requires rousing inventiveness. Dreaming a reality that holds space for all our intersectional bodyminds is how we declare ourselves in a world that, as Audre Lorde writes, "we were never meant to survive." This type of creativity is sacred and generative, and it is informed by Gloria Anzaldúa's description of imagination. In her book *Light in the Dark/Luz en lo Oscuro*, she writes, "Imagination opens the road to both personal and societal change—transformation of self, consciousness, community, culture, society."[38] Imagination is how we change our individual and collective perspectives and move toward liberation.[39] I think about Patty and Leroy's crip-dreaming of Sins Invalid through a similar lens: imagination is how they began to manifest a world where disabled, queer, gender-nonconforming, and trans bodyminds of color were embraced in accessible, revolutionary love.

Sins Invalid outlines their vision and mission statement on their website, sinsinvalid dot org. Their vision extends their radical imagining by conceptualizing possibilities and futures where we, in all our intersectional glories, are valued and whole:

> Sins Invalid recognizes that we will be liberated as whole beings—as disabled, as queer, as brown, as black, as gender non-conforming, as trans, as women, as men, as non-binary gendered—we are far greater whole than partitioned. We recognize that our allies emerge from many communities and that demographic identity alone does not determine one's commitment to liberation. Sins Invalid is committed to social and economic justice for all people with disabilities ... moving beyond individual legal rights to collective human rights. Our stories, embedded in analysis, offer

paths from identity politics to unity amongst all oppressed people, laying a foundation for a collective claim of liberation and beauty.

This statement stays true to Sins Invalid's original intent of dreaming, enacting, and practicing disabled, queer of color recognition and wholeness. Grounded in the fifth principle of Disability Justice, wholeness advocates that disabled bodyminds are not defective, incomplete, or lacking, as the medical model of disability would have us believe. This principle unsettles how we define wholeness from ableist and capitalist synonyms like productivity and success and instead asks us to crip, queer, and decolonize wholeness. This principle tells us that we do not need to meet a capitalist benchmark of success to be viewed as important. We are whole and valuable simply because we are ourselves. Sins Invalid's vision that "we will be liberated as whole beings" reframes wholeness as a liberatory practice of diverse bodymind celebration.

The stories and historical retellings that come from this place of cripped wholeness also embed self-love practices within them. I use "self-love" throughout the book in the way that author and poet Sonya Renee Taylor crafts it: self-love is the radical politics of embodiment and loving. In her book *The Body Is Not an Apology*, Sonya writes that radical self-love is the realization that "We did not start life in a negative partnership with our bodies",[40] that "Radical self-love is indeed our inherent natural state, but social, political, and economic systems of oppression have distanced us from that knowing."[41] When I dream of what intrinsically disabled, queer of color wholeness looks like, when I ground myself in Sins Invalid's vision, I find a performance project that seeks to create space and art-activism that invites us back into our whole selves, just as we are. It is an invitation to return and plant seeds of change-making.

To grow distant from the self, to erase parts of ourselves, is, to use Sonya's language, to live in "negative partnership" with our bodyminds. This distancing is akin to ableism, racism, and cis-heteropatriarchy's erasure. In this distancing, we are made invisible and distant from ourselves so that we are no longer whole, radiant beings. To ground Sins Invalid in the vision that disabled, queer of color bodyminds deserve to be seen in all of their identities and in all of their beauty requires an amplification of radical self-love and wholeness; it requires a movement away from the negative, toxic bodymind partnerships that this world and all of its intersecting oppressions have forced upon us. When I spoke with Patty, she/they advised that all our disabled, queer of color bodyminds deserve to be seen and that this practice begins with ourselves: "At a certain point, we all need to make a choice about living … I can't erase myself. I can't participate in my own erasure."[42] It is integral to Disability Justice and Sins Invalid that we actively make ourselves known, wholly and radically, to ourselves once again.

—————

The commitment to visibility, recognition, and communal love and liberation continues in Sins Invalid's mission statement. They begin by emphasizing the importance of community: "Sins Invalid is a disability justice-based performance project that incubates and celebrates artists with disabilities, centralizing artists of color and LGBT/gender-variant artists as communities who have been historically marginalized. Led by disabled people of color, Sins Invalid's performance work explores the themes of sexuality, embodiment and the disabled body, developing provocative work where paradigms of 'normal' and 'sexy' are challenged, offering instead a vision of beauty and sexuality inclusive of all bodies and communities."

Sins Invalid intentionally supports the disabled many who have been excluded from the mainstream Disability Rights Movement and from nondisabled social justice spaces. Their disabled, queer of color dreaming has led to this place of expansion and possibility.[43] Here, they teach us not simply how to unlearn ableism's oppressions, but rather, they teach us how to trouble and rewrite ableist, racist, and cis-heteropatriarchal paradigms that shift who we can view as "normal" and "sexy." For Sins Invalid, embodiment and beauty are not stagnant things; they are luminescent and always changing.

Patty and I first spoke in 2014 about Sins Invalid and its centering of disabled, queer of color community. She/they explained that it is critical that this art-activism, this dream-making, be led by those most impacted by ableism, racism, and cis-heteropatriarchy: "[Sins Invalid is] not about somebody else. It's not an organization doing something about other people. It's about us. It's about our experiences as disabled people, as queer folks with disabilities, and as gender non-conforming people with disabilities."[44] This centering aligns itself with Disability Justice's second principle: the leadership of the most impacted. This principle argues that "We know ableism exists in the context of other historical systematic oppressions. We know to truly have liberation we must be led by those who know the most about these systems and how they work."[45] Those most impacted by oppression carry within them the knowledge to empower change and the potential to dream us forward toward revolution. By enacting the leadership of the most impacted, Sins Invalid actualizes intentional space for the collective wisdom of intersectional communities that have long been ignored and devalued.

Patty remembers that Sins Invalid's first performance in 2006 was an important communal antidote for crip erasure. Named *From Sacrificed to Sacred*, the evening took place at the Brava Theater in San Francisco's Mission District. As a theater that promotes and supports art made by underrepresented communities, the Brava was an ideal first location. For Patty, the performance became a reminder that despite the world's persistent and systemic social and political disposability of our body-minds, disabled, queer of color communities exist. We, the many, are resilient and we refuse the forced legacy of crip isolation and institutionalization.[46] Disabled community members joined together at the Brava with friends, on their own, and with their personal assistants to experience what a thriving disabled, queer of color imagination could create. Within the walls of the theater that night, a crip-centric liberated zone grew among everyone's collective refusal to live, work, and love in an ableist, racist, cis-heteropatriarchal culture that limits our access and our understandings of beauty and sexuality.

Reflecting on that night, Patty writes, "when the lights went down and a hush went through the audience, the magic unfolded. Three hundred people witnessed disabled artist after disabled artist, talking about desire, displaying our bodies and doing it in a way where *we* were setting the terms of engagement. We moved the audience through a new paradigm, with emotions in the theater shifting from voyeuristic eroticism to intimacy to loss to anger to risk to aroused by a new vision of embodiment."[47]

Crip persistence is the "magic" that Patty witnessed that first night, a night that would result in over a decade of art-activism. Crip persistence took stage at the Brava and reminded a diverse audience of three hundred people that willfully self-crafted possibility exists outside of all the regulatory lessons we have been taught. Beyond the medicalization of our bodies as defect and lack, we are, as disability studies scholar Eli Clare writes, "brilliant imperfections." We, in all our luster, carry within us the potential to forge new, radical, loving worlds. We can and do thrive beyond normativity and all of its overwhelming oppressions.

Naming Us Home

When Patty and Leroy searched for a name for the performance project, they arrived at *Sins Invalid: An Unshamed Claim to Beauty in the Face of Invisibility*. Patty and Leroy reveal that the name evokes the eugenics and morality-based narratives that have for so long normalized the ways we think about disability. As a word and a concept, "invalid" carries heavy on its back the lineage of eugenics, when disabled and ill bodyminds were labeled as unfit, deviant, and undesirable. It reminds us of all the people who were forcibly sterilized in the 1920s onward, beginning with *Buck v. Bell*, the landmark case in 1927 when US Supreme Court Justice Oliver Wendell Holmes Jr. approved a Virginia state statute to legally perform sterilizations on institutionalized men and women without their consent. *Invalid* reminds us of how disabled people were, and still are, viewed as being unworthy of procreation; sometimes, we are viewed as unworthy of living.[48]

Just like any other word, *invalid* slip-shifts in meaning depending on context and who interprets it. Patty shares that sometimes people pronounce *invalid* as in-VUH-lid, a word with ableist roots of its own. At other times, for Patty the word reflects the restrictive and ableist rules of our capitalist culture: we are only worthy if we contribute to capitalism in the ways capitalism demands.[49]

The second half of their name, *sins*, also holds expansive meaning. On the one hand, to say that disabilities are the result of sin is an old myth. Often labeled the religious moral model of disability, this model argues that a child's disability is a penalty for parental immorality.[50] As an extension of or synonym for disability, the moral model teaches us that our disabled bodyminds are a transgression and that we are a regret, that it would be best if we were institutionalized, warehoused in a nursing home, or if our disabilities stayed family secrets never to be spoken of again. On the other hand, the concept of *sin* can also be applied to queerness, an identity that many institutions like family, religion, and medicine have taught us is shameful and abnormal. When exploring another branch connected to this religious root, sinning also relates to the act of having sex and perhaps even to the unthinkability of crip sex.[51] *Sin* can refer to who we are, how we move through this world, and who we love just as much as it can refer to the fact that we are alive and that we exist.

To invalidate *sins* is to imagine a new reality altogether. Sins Invalid generates a political ripeness of persistence and disobedience, lessons that Sara Ahmed applies to feminist killjoys and that I extend here to disabled, queer of color rebels.[52] Sins Invalid teaches us that our existence as disabled, queer of color bodyminds must always be unapologetic; it must be "an unshamed claim," something that we can firmly and proudly stake our futures on. We refuse to fit into the normalcy that ableism, racism, cis-heteropatriarchy and all the oppressive, intersecting networks dictate. This refusal results in what Sara calls persistence and disobedience: "Mere persistence can be an act of disobedience. And then: you have to persist in being disobedient. And then: to exist is disobedient."[53] Sins Invalid is a rallying cry, a crip call to a community that has been taught that obedience means performing nondisability, whiteness, and cis-heteropatriarchy. Our communities have been taught that our stories of bodymind rebellion and protest against nondisabled supremacy are inconvenient if they do not align with narratives of tragedy, of overcoming, of pity, or of inspiration porn.[54] We have been taught that our desires, our sexualities, and our beauty are not valid if we are disabled, if we are fat, if we are people of color, if we are bold with our gender nonconformity and queerness.

In their name and in their practice, Sins Invalid helps us to remember that our bodymind existence is never intrusive or sinful. This world fiercely needs our disabled, queer of color bodymind disobedience. In the coming pages, the performance project shows us that, in fact, we have survived the world's attempt to erase us because of our communal disabled, queer of color disobedience. We have survived because we have crafted crip-centric liberated zones where shame is undone from who we are. *Sins Invalid*: our stories, our solidarity, and our creation, in all their revolutionary potentials, have home in this name.

———

By politicizing disabled, queer of color artmaking and Disability Justice activism, Sins Invalid challenges our mandated obedience, the bodymind compromises that our everyday forces us to make. They invalidate the desexualization and medicalization that we are forced to edge up against. In this new, disobedient, unapologetic reality, our disabled, queer of color bodyminds become beauty amplified.

CHAPTER 2

Creating Crip-Centric Liberated Zones

A crip-centric liberated zone is a multidirectional community love practice. It is a place of our own creation where we, the disabled, queer of color many, can exist and thrive liberated from the oppressions that relegate our daily lives. When directed inward, the love practice of a crip-centric liberated zone gifts us with strategies for re-centering and decolonizing our bodyminds. When directed outward, the zone politically transforms the places we inhabit—even if temporarily—into hubs of communal bodymind witnessing.

Patty introduced me to this phrase during our interview in April 2018. She/they shared that in crip-centric liberated zones, we persist, grow, and feel relief. The crip-centric liberated zone's love practice grounds us in the reality and gut knowing that our bodyminds belong, despite the world's insistence on erasing us. Centering cripness in such a space reminds us of the need for cross movement solidarity, for collective resistance, and for the unwavering valuing of our bodyminds. It is an acknowledgment of all that Disability Justice enacts. When our world persists in Othering disabled, queer of color communities and their experiences, crip-centric liberated zones center communal resilience and our collective practice of becoming.

For Crip-Centric Liberated Zones, You Need Disability Justice

Crip-centric liberated zones aim to heal and hold transformative space for all our bodyminds. When I began imagining what a place like this would do and how it would function, I kept arriving to the somatic, to embodied reactions. I thought of how, at many points in my life, I felt like I was holding back parts of myself to the point of breakage. My body-mind recalls two moments here. One is associated with my queerness, the other with my Madness. I remember how the pressure and weight of culture and family buried my queerness and how, after a while, it became absence and void. Madness occupied a similar sensation. I did not think I could professionally disclose without risking a bombardment of stereotypes, without being reduced in all the toxic ways that nondisabled supremacy and sanism reduce the Mad. Anyone who has had to swallow parts of themselves knows how this causes bodymind wreckage, how it causes loss, and how it distances us from ourselves. I also remember how disclosure and naming my Mad queer bodymind felt like breakage of another kind: a joyous explosion, a liberation of feelings. I remember that I arrived at this place of abundance and rootedness because I had found my disabled, queer of color community.

Although I did not have the language for it then, I had found myself in a crip-centric liberated zone, a place where I could take up space, where I could break open and be seen and held in community as my truest self. My bodymind remembers the journey now as I write this, and I am more aware that just as much as crip-centric liberated zones can be locations, they can also be a cultivation of feeling and experience; they can be found on blog posts, during workshops or webinars, or on websites. They can thrive in our bedrooms and on our computer screens when no one else is around. Because so many of us still enter into spaces that force us to select one identity while casting the others aside, because so many of us are still searching for spaces liberated from ableism, racism, and cis-heteropatriarchy, often these zones are temporary and are generated out of necessity.

The Disability Justice principles of collective access and collective liberation inform crip-centric liberated zones. As a foundational principle, collective access advocates that spaces and events can push past ableism and instead creatively establish access for all our bodyminds.[55] As Sins Invalid grew and began to host more performances and more workshops, collective access manifested as a consideration of diverse disabilities as well as gender and sexual identities, embodiments, and class backgrounds. To construct a place supported by collective access where we can share our bodymind needs without shame or hesitation moves all of us toward a collective liberation "that leaves no bodymind behind."[56]

However temporary Sins Invalid's crip-centric liberated zones are, they offer respite. Their performances are a good example of what collective access looks like, how it functions, and why it is such a crucial part of collective liberation. Yes, Sins Invalid offers American Sign Language (ASL) interpreters and wheelchair accessibility, but they also ensure access to gender-neutral restrooms and seating for audience members who might need extra space for their bodies. They provide language options as well as audio descriptions. They remind audience members that they are entering scent-free venues and that low-stimulation quiet spaces are available for decompression. Lastly, tickets are often available on a sliding scale basis, and no one is ever turned away for a lack of funds. These intentional and expansive examples of what cripped, queered, anti-capitalist access can look like illustrate the crip-centric liberated zones that Disability Justice as practice and process facilitates.

––––––––––

When I saw Sins Invalid perform at the ODC Theater in 2016, I felt the recognition of community and again, an ecstatic breakage, a bodymind opening and welcoming. In the low-stimulation room, my Mad mind was as calm as it could be in a new environment and my needs were met without justification. Community educator and organizer Mia Mingus names this feeling "access intimacy." It is "that elusive, hard to describe feeling when someone else 'gets' your access needs ... ground-level, with no need for explanations."[57] Most importantly, Mia argues that access intimacy "can transform ordinary access into a tool for liberation."[58] Although no one space can be completely accessible to everyone present, Sins Invalid's intentional creation of collective access is the closest thing many of us have ever experienced. Crip-centric liberated zones serve as transitory spaces where we are made familiar to ourselves once again and where we are re-centered in the power and potential of our bodyminds.

––––––––––

Decolonizing Our Bodyminds and
Our Communities for Liberation

Perhaps one of the most generative parts of crip-centric liberated zones are the ways they invite us to integrate the temporary liberation we experience into our everyday lives and communities. After we leave the performance or the workshop, the space of disabled, queer of color deliverance, how can we too continue in our Disability Justice dreaming, movement building, and culture work? How can we envision the "yet-to-be map"[59] of Disability Justice and collective liberation in our communal and home spaces? When Patty and I spoke in 2018 about the different ways we can protest the ableist framings of our bodyminds, she/they foregrounded decolonization as the foundation of this work. Educator Nina Asher describes colonization as destruction, as a power imbalance that causes the "dislocation, disembodiment, and objectification"[60] of communities of color.[61] To begin to undo this intergenerational practice of dislocation and disembodiment, we must begin to revise the ways colonization and ableism create systematic occupations and exploitations of the land, [62] of our bodyminds, and of the bodies of those who live on the land.[63] If we can begin to do this, if we can learn how to decolonize ourselves, then we can learn to reclaim our histories of resilience and resistance.

At the University of California, Berkeley's Disability Incarcerated Symposium in 2015, Sins Invalid organized a performance event and participatory altar called *Disability Liberated*.[64] Here, writer, healer, activist, and Sins Invalid artist Aurora Levins Morales read "Disability Liberated," a poem that identifies the entwined history of ableism and colonization. When I think about how crip-centric liberated zones teach us to decolonize our disabled bodyminds, I think of this poem. Poems, too, can be liberated zones, places we inhabit when we read, and when our reading spills over into the lives we actualize:

> Our history is in our bodies. And these are the sterilized multitudes, women of Puerto Rico, one out of three, migrant worker mothers in labor told to sign what they can't read, the poverty-stricken, the weak limbed, the feebleminded, the queer, a poor girl from Virginia, deemed too stupid to breed, the ones who get migraines, or drink, or like sex, dark skinned, immigrant, colonized, Jew, people like me, people like you ... strapped down under surgeons' knives, their bloodlines severed, their children disappeared by stone faced people desperately building a master race to rule the world. Yet here we are, and here we are fruitful, our stories flower, take wing, reproduce like windblown seeds.

This poem locates us in an embodied history of disabled communities of color that are often left untold. We cannot talk about ableism, nor can we address it without acknowledging this gap. Aurora names the history of the disabled, many of whom were unwillingly sterilized, institutionalized, and forcibly turned into "clinical material."[65] The poem "Disability Liberated" is the story of disabled people of color who were disembodied and objectified, disabled people of color who were dehumanized and colonized.

To witness—or for the first time learn—the retelling of this history is the first step toward decolonizing our present and creating a crip-centric liberated zone for all disabled, queer of color bodyminds. We need to know the experiences and stories of our disabled ancestors of color if we are to create a space where we can celebrate our multiple identities and progress Disability Justice forward. We need to know, as

Aurora writes, that our ancestral history is *in* our bodyminds. For Patty, this performance becomes one of the many ways we can apply this practice of decolonization so that we can once again re-know ourselves outside of the alienating frameworks of colonialism and ableism.[66]

———

I am finding more and more that for Sins Invalid, to engage in the deco-lonial project of crip-centric liberated zones is to be in recognition of unspoken crip pasts. In an interview with the *American Quarterly*, Patty spoke about *Disability Liberated*. In particular, she/they discussed the importance of when cultural work and performance bears witness: "That's important in all of Sins Invalid's work: to try to bring people into the room who aren't there. It's clear how that's demonstrating a resistant politic and bearing witness to the current conditions of abuse, but also acknowledging the humanity of those who have died and their move-ment toward being our ancestors."[67]

Sins Invalid resists the lengthy history of forcibly relegating disabled bodyminds to state-supported institutions, segregated schools, and nursing homes. They resist the ableist, capitalist legacy of seclusion, abuse, and neglect; they resist the legacy of intentional forgetting. Although they weave remembering into their activism, performances, and workshops, *Disability Liberated* particularly holds space for those in our communities who are incarcerated and institutionalized.

Sins Invalid describes the event and altar as "a furious elegy paying homage to the countless disabled lives that have been lost to the vio-lence of able-bodied supremacy incarceration, policing and institu-tionalization."[68] During the performance, we gain access into the lives of communities that are often isolated from the nondisabled majority:

a phone call from an incarcerated, paraplegic woman at the Richard J. Donovan Correctional Facility in San Diego; a story of children on a hospital ward supporting each other, resilient; exhausted faces of people looking up at the ceiling, down at the floor, and out of the institution's window; a small voice in the dark saying, "I am here. I am caught." It is an act of decolonial remembering to highlight these narratives. It is the creation of a crip-centric liberated zone that emphasizes our collective, disabled, queer of color need for honoring the many we have lost and the many we must continue to advocate for. This is liberation from all the systems of oppression with which our lives intersect. This is breathing, again.

———————

Healing Ourselves Whole

As a location, experience, and moment, crip-centric liberated zones and their Disability Justice practice give the disabled, queer of color many the tools needed for bodymind celebration and healing. When in community, we feel our way back to ourselves and away from the ableist belief that we are inherently broken and unworthy of celebration or love.

For many of us, Sins Invalid is a first. It is the first time we are in a queer, mixed ability space of color. It is the first time we have access to a low-stimulation room during an event, the first time we have accessible, roomy seating for our bodies. Sometimes, it is the first time we see other folks that look like us. Writer, cultural worker, artist-activist, and Sins Invalid community member Leah Lakshmi Piepzna-Samarasinha (she/they) explained to me her/their first experience at a Sins Invalid performance this way:

The first thing I noticed was the audience. I had never seen an audience like that before ... there were so many disabled people ... there were so many people using different adaptive devices. I was going on a night where there was ASL interpretations so there were like a ton of Deaf folks and hard of hearing folks ... there were people who were stimming, people who were using MCS masks ... and people who were so queer and so trans and so black and so brown all at once ... It changed my world to see that that was a community that was possible. I had never seen that, never.[69]

Leah's description identifies another important gift of crip-centric liberated zones: recognition, validation, and healing. Serving as zones for liberation, Sins Invalid's performances communicate not only that disabled, queer of color bodyminds exist, but beyond that, that they are active storytellers, meaning makers, and artist-activists that cultivate collective liberation together.

Patty and I spoke in greater detail about the healing impact of the recognition that takes place during a Sins Invalid event. She/they shared that much of it has to do with being witnessed by community. I think of the word "witness" here, beyond the definition as an act of observation or a moment of bearing testimony. Witness is also "evidence; proof"; witness is also "confirmation."[70] In the crip-centric liberated zones Sins Invalid creates, we see—in all the diverse ways we "see"—one another. We witness, and we are witnessed by our communities. Power comes from seeing your communities on stage, in a documentary, or leading a workshop; it comes from experiencing stories about disabled body-minds that center lust, attraction, and playfulness, that tell more than the master narratives of trauma, tragedy, cure, and overcoming that are so often inscribed onto us. Being seen, whether in person or while online, is how we create the visibility and love that is so integral to collective liberation. Patty advised that these spaces are not just transformational for the audience. The healing and feelings of resilience also take place for the Sins Invalid performers and crew: "Some say it feels like church."[71]

I think about this phrase, this feeling. I have never been to church, so I roll this metaphor around on my tongue. I imagine a crip church as a place where all our bodyminds are welcomed and not questioned. Thinking of crip-centric liberated zones, of the ways they decolonize and create room for us to live and breathe resistant to the intersecting oppressions that regulate our every day, if only for a few hours, I envision embrace, appreciation, and bodymind consideration as locations, as places we can visit. This is my anti-colonial, anti-patriarchal, non-divisive version of church, and maybe for some of us, this is the space that Sins Invalid holds.

For me, attending live Sins Invalid performances and viewing recordings online in the dark of my bedroom felt, instead, like a door opening, like a greeting. I was introduced to a radical and political possibility that I had yet to dream for myself. It was my first introduction to Disability Justice. It was the first time I ever saw the beautiful, rebellious potential of disabled bodyminds outside all of the ableist and sanist messages I had been taught about my own community and myself. It was the first of so many things.

Surviving COVID-19,
Embracing Crip-Centric Liberated Zones

As I write this chapter, we are in the middle of a global pandemic. I live in Pomona, a predominately working class, Latinx city on the edge of Los Angeles County, and right now in California, we are experiencing an extreme resurgence of positive COVID-19 cases. I end this chapter by focusing on crip-centric liberated zones and how their practice of enacting mutual aid and care networks now enters into our everyday, so much so that nondisabled folks are learning what these words mean and why they are so critical for the survival of all our bodyminds.

I return to the medicine that is Leah's *Care Work* for definitions and guidance. She/they define mutual aid[72] as a coming together of disabled and nondisabled communities for the purpose of supporting one another outside of a charity model.[73] She/they write that "Mutual aid, as opposed to charity, does not connote moral superiority of the giver over the receiver. White people didn't invent the concept of mutual aid— many precolonial (and after) Black, Indigenous, and brown communities have complex webs of exchanges of care."[74] Rebel Sidney Black, a light-skinned multiracial, nonbinary, disabled community organizer, extends this definition by acknowledging that many of us already engage in diverse practices of mutual aid:

> Mutual aid is that random person from the internet bringing a hot meal when you can't get out of bed, it's cleaning or spiritually cleansing the home of someone who's too severely depressed to do it themselves, it's staying up late talking to that suicidal friend, helping unpack an apartment after someone moves, giving rides to chemo, visiting or writing letters to folks in prison, walking someone's dogs when they can't walk

[themselves]. It can also look like sharing coping skills, survival skills, job search skills. Mutual aid can be sharing medicine, making medicine, helping sift through allopathic doctors to find a good fit, or referring someone to that awesome working-class naturopath you know.[75]

This description clearly frames mutual aid as a non-hierarchal and anti-capitalist structure of giving, of tenderness, and of cripped care. With so many out of work because of COVID-19, many more communities are now, for the first time, calling on mutual aid and its constant focus on collaboration.[76] Community members who were still earning a paycheck while working from home engaged in campaigns to disperse the stimulus checks they received from the government to community members.[77] Only people with a social security number were given checks, and yet for collective liberation, our communities know that everyone needs and deserves emergency relief funds. Folks are donating food and resource sharing ways to access free food; they are creating community refrigerators and pantries[78] and giving laptops and hotspots to families and students who are trying to navigate distance learning and working from home.

The practice of collaboration, care, and organizing has also resulted in knowledge archiving and sharing. Social justice collectives and mutual aid networks such as Disability Justice Culture Club, Mutual Aid Medford and Somerville (MAMAS), and the Audre Lorde Project, among many others, have committed themselves to sharing resources online, particularly for disabled, queer of color communities.[79] Leah created the Google Doc "Half Assed Disabled Prepper Tips for Preparing for a Coronavirus Quarantine," and disabled fat folks of color led by Fat Rose/Fat Lib Ink created the "Fat-Assed Prepper Survival Tips for

Preparing for a Coronavirus Quarantine," a resource sharing guide and mutual aid support system.

These responses encourage us to remember that our disabled, queer of color knowledge is alchemy; it is community medicine by us and for us, and now, nondisabled folks are paying notice to concepts long practiced in disability communities: mutual aid, accessibility, and pod mapping—Mia Mingus's term for a tool that helps to map out small communities of accountability and care. Our knowledge and implementation of mutual aid demonstrates that crip-centric liberated zones can transform us into intersecting, supportive, communal systems. In this place, actions that are not monetized carry collective significance. There is crip-centric liberatory power in getting groceries for a friend, in watering someone's garden, in collecting and sharing resources online, in holding e-space with community members who are grieving. We will continue to grow forward accessibly and lovingly by practicing skill sharing, crowdsourcing knowledge, and cultivating mutual aid resources. In crowdsourcing mutual aid resources, we are also cripping[80] and crowdsourcing care.

In all the incredible ways we are healing and sustaining our communities during the COVID-19 pandemic, we also need to remember to turn inward and work to restore ourselves. In April 2020, Sins Invalid shared a blog post entitled, "Show Your Cripself that You Are Loved." The post includes what they call "grounded support": "We've watched/read/ heard so much information about the Novel Coronavirus—And most of it has made us more anxious and less grounded. We want to offer folks a little bit of grounded support."[81] The energy and goal setting of what is generated in crip-centric liberated zones infuses Sins Invalid's affirmations and targeted ways of engaging with the community.

They begin the blog by grounding us in our glorious bodymind realities: "You are the only person that can offer what only you can offer to the world, in all of history and from this moment onward ... Your bodymind deserves care. You always have, you do now, and You always will deserve care."[82] As I read and reread these messages, I moved toward wholeness, bodymind love, and consideration. Returning to the original definition of crip-centric liberated zones as a multidirectional community love practice, I read these affirmations as a reminder that to give to our communities, we must also give to our bodyminds and liberate ourselves. We must slow down, rest, nourish, and take care.

Although the second half of the post includes questions and prompts rooted in mutual aid practices and in pod mapping, the following list by Sins Invalid offers an abbreviated, workable point of entry:

- Which principles of Disability Justice can support you while you navigate through your response to coronavirus?
- We know lots of disabled people have recently lost their income/ resources. Can you look through 2 (two) of these links to see if they can support you?
- How does your brilliance shine, even in a global pandemic?
- Knowing that much of the world does not have access to digital communication or Internet access, who is one person you can reach out to, breaking through the isolation for a disabled person?
- Now that non-disabled people have experienced the effect of isolation and lack of access first hand, name two people that you can have conversations with about being a better ally to you when you can't leave the house.[83]

At times, I have found myself overwhelmed with the abundance of pandemic survival information and community organizing. For anyone who similarly finds themselves in this place and is in search of user-friendly guidance, these prompts offer tangible, accessible ways of creating communal and internal liberated zones that remind us of the knowledges, histories, and strategies of endurance that we carry: we hold the awareness and consideration needed to support our bodyminds and our communities. With our Disability Justice resistance vocabulary and practice, with our recognition of what crip-centric liberated zones bring, we can begin to flourish forward and bring on our fiercest disabled, queer of color imaginings.

CHAPTER 3

In Love and Community, Like the Trees

My wife was the first person to tell me about the sequoias and their adaptability. She was the first person to tell me about their expansive network of connectivity and their intertwined root systems. As we stood there among them, our hands reaching out to touch the moss and bark, I imagined an elder community with outstretched arms, fingers grasping, holding, and giving. I began to think of what it means to center the knowledge of trees.

I begin here, in this place of earth and connection, because this is where Patty Berne led me when we spoke over Zoom about the challenges that culminated in moments of growth and transformation for Sins Invalid. Informed and guided by Disability Justice, even in its creation of crip-centric liberated zones and its imagining of disabled, queer of color resilience, Sins Invalid, like any other organization, has had growing pains. Perhaps unlike other performance projects, their remedy is a love practice.

"Indeed, all great movements for social justice in our society have strongly emphasized a love ethic."

In August 2020, Patty shared with me that Sins Invalid's practice of Disability Justice is intentional. The performance project doesn't simply engage with the political framework. Disability Justice becomes how they create, how they work, and also how they grow; this practice has everything to do with love. As the performance project developed, Patty said that she/they often asked, and continue to ask, "Am I practicing love?" For Patty and Sins Invalid, love for self and love for community are acts that require continual self-inquiry. In this process of questions and examinations, the performance project has found that as accessible as they try to make their events and the spaces they inhabit, sometimes the goal of achieving collective access falls short:

> The reality is that we do Disability Justice work, but we are doing this work in real time. [Sometimes our goals are aspirational]. Sometimes we might end up working with a white interpreter or a transcription service not based in the U.S., but [who can do the work] faster when we need something done quickly … At a party, an intern was saying that the event wasn't very accessible for people that are neurodivergent …. We try, but there are compromises we make, and we don't execute things perfectly because we are human, and we are living and working in systems of oppression.

It is a manifestation of crip love to actively self-inquire and scrutinize organizational practices. Sins Invalid realizes that as humans engaging in cross-disability organizing, they are not going to get everything right a hundred percent of the time: there will be moments of forgetting, best practices that don't consider the needs of all bodyminds, and gaps in funding –in our capitalist system, access costs money—and things are going to get messy. These moments of reflection and the repetition of the question, "Am I practicing love?" cautions Patty and fellow organizers that they must continue to question their decisions and directions.

———————

After Patty and I ended our conversation, I reread bell hooks's writings on love, particularly from her book *All About Love: New Visions*. bell hooks renders love a verb, what she calls a "transformative force."[84] Early on in the book, she connects love and social justice work so that an enactment of love becomes a critical component in maintaining and extending the actions of activist communities. She writes, "Indeed, all the great movements for social justice in our society have strongly emphasized a love ethic."[85] bell hooks connects her love ethics to freedom and liberation. Love as a transformative force charges us to challenge and question systems of oppression; love is how we get free.[86] Patty's constant questioning—am I practicing love?—attempts to interrogate the practices of the performance project: what can be done better? What harms are we causing and how can we remedy them? This self-inquiry and recognition, this drive to always do better, is an extension of love ethics. It is the remembrance that we must always be "in service" to our communities if we are to move toward collective liberation and freedom.[87]

———————

Patty also stressed that compassion is an intrinsic part of a love practice: "The most important thing is, like with any relationship, that we are compassionate toward ourselves and toward other people when we are in an aspirational place." To dream crip, queer, decolonial dreams in our ableist, racist, cis-heteropatriarchal world demands self and communal compassion. This kind of dreaming, this kind of aspirational work, comes with large doses of good intentions and moments of slippage and miscalculations. For Patty, compassion gives us permission to pause and investigate our own internalized oppressions. We can give ourselves the permission to look lovingly and expansively beyond the moment to discover what we need to change and what we need to develop the next time around. Compassion is the tool we need in our disabled, queer of color communities as we build relationships with one another toward revolution.

"If we can't respect one another, how are we going to be in alliance with each other?"

During Sins Invalid's decade-long existence of community interaction, Patty disclosed that the performance project has, without intending to, caused hurt:

> We've engaged with dozens of people in substantive ways over the years. It's a small group of people but there definitely have been people who felt unseen, not listened to, and are just done and honestly that's what hurts the most. The first time that happened I felt like I should quit, like I was a giant fuck up; I hurt someone and that is the opposite purpose of why I started Sins. It took a lot for Leroy and I to metabolize: yes someone is hurt, they have a valid right, and as an organization we have to do better next time.

Patty's emphasis of accountability here resonates. It is the broaching of difficult topics, of acknowledging harm, and of developing new ways to move forward collectively after all the changes have been made. The respect and love they have for their communities are what initiate Patty and Leroy's desire to metabolize hurt: "If we can't respect one another, how are we going to be in alliance with each other?" Metabolizing in this way, in a culture of inquiry and respect, is how networks of solidarity and interconnectivity are made and how harms are reconciled.

Even though much of our talk focused on Sins Invalid, Patty stressed that the self must also be included in conversations of respect, alliance, and love. This topic came up for Patty when she/they reflected on the administrative work she/they do:

> As a woman of color, I was trying to support the access needs of [a white, cis heterosexual man], but I didn't realize the way I was playing into the invisibilization of labor that a woman of color typically provides. The way we do a lot of the emotional labor or the way we do a lot of the unseen administrative work, the low-profile things, the unglamorous parts of an organization right, administrative stuff, the nuts and the bolts. And most admin people aren't recognized, unfortunately, when they are a critical part of the organization. To write things down, to document, and to make agendas; there is power in that too. And I let my labor become invisible and that really reinforced my internalized sexism.

Despite the contributions of women, gender nonconforming, and trans people of color in activist movements, in our communities, and in our familial spaces and workspaces, patriarchy and white supremacy continue to exploit and invisibilize the labor of women of color. Patty's experience exhibits how gendered and racialized oppressions impact the workplace, especially when they are internalized.

_____

One of Sins Invalid's growing pains involves a process of unlearning. In the creation of crip-centric liberated zones, in the aspirational creation of spaces that honor collective access, everyone involved in the performance project must engage in self-inquiry. Everyone must engage in the difficult, tangled, and often repetitive process of unlearning the systems of oppression that they bring with them to the performance project. Patty adds that this process was, for both her/them and others, complicated specifically because of the liberatory community Sins Invalid commits to constructing: "What I want to say is that we are an organization that has multiple intersections around race and gender, sexuality, class, education, access, and disability and so because of that, there are so many things we can internalize and there are so many ways we can bump heads. Because we have a really high-level of trust and love, sometimes those oppressions don't get noted because we are not clocking [them] and our defenses are down."

The remedy here for Patty is to enact the glorious, imperfect messiness that is Disability Justice and its intersectional focus. It is remembering that we all have been raised in what bell hooks calls "a system of domination," a system that resists the journey toward freedom and liberation. When practicing a love ethic, opportunities for new growth and strengthening can arise. Realizing that she/they were participating in the invisibilizing of her/their own work resulted in a powerful conversation wherein Patty acknowledged her/their feelings and the harm she/they were experiencing; it resulted in a creation of boundaries. This is a decolonial practice, an awareness based in courage, compassion, inquiry, and above all, love.

bell hooks writes about the decolonizing that happens in moments of self-inquiry and questioning this way: "Whenever those of us who are members of exploited and oppressed groups dare to critically interrogate our locations, the identities and allegiances that inform how we live out our lives, we begin the process of decolonization. If we discover in ourselves self-hatred, low self-esteem, or internalized white supremacist thinking and we face it, we can begin to heal. Acknowledging the truth of our reality, both individual and collective, is a necessary stage for personal and political growth."[88]

It is a radical shift to think of self-transformation and self-inquiry as decolonial practice, as love practice, and as a way to move us all toward collective liberation. Anytime an intersectional community comes together to create change that reframes ableist, racist, cis-heteropatriarchal, and capitalist ideals, internal and collective adjustments are needed. Although, as Patty notes, this process may sometimes take longer to broach depending on the dynamic, self and communal inquiry and awareness are a crucial part of building meaningful and supportive networks of connection and love.

"We have to model our crip networks after the billions of fungi."

During our Zoom call, Patty's attendant comes in and out of the frame. They are helping Patty get ready for the day, adorning her/them with jewelry, and combing and parting her/their damp hair. Halfway through the conversation, tea with boba arrives and an outstretched arm holding the chilled cup draws toward Patty's mouth. As the conversation shifts to the interconnectivity of love and community, I can't help but notice that what Patty is talking about is unfolding right in front of me.

She/they begin with a story: "I was recently listening to an audiobook called *The Hidden Life of Trees* [by Peter Wohlleben] and learned that trees live in community. They are connected through their root systems and through scent … They can look out for each other. Shouldn't we all do that?" Patty describes a reciprocal community, a coordinated love place dedicated to the revolutionary potentials of care and interdependence. I nod, listening as Patty's attendant creates two perfect buns of hair, one on either side of her/their head. Patty continues: "We have to model our crip networks after the billions of fungi; the mycelium network has the ability to communicate and support each other beyond what we [as humans] have demonstrated so far; I think we can strive for that."

After our talk, I look up "mycelium." I learn that these "thread-like structures of fungi" grow underground. Mycelia are root-like, delicate, and expansive. They break down, absorb, and share nutrients with nearby plants; they gain strength by being in community with one another. The more I read, the more I begin to think of words like stabilize, support, and nourish. I begin to understand Patty's metaphor.

———————

It has been a week since Patty and I spoke on Zoom and through thinking about interconnectivity, I reexplore author and activist adrienne maree brown's book, *Emergent Strategy*. For adrienne, the natural world around us can teach us strategies of survival and resilience. In the natural world, we can create transformative change through small interactions. She references the migrating knowledge of starlings and their flock, the knowledge of ants, and the communal lessons of mycelium and trees. With all of these examples, adrienne emphasizes the sustainability, adaptability, collective leadership, and trust that nature teaches us. She asks us to consider the nature lessons we can learn and then apply to our organizing work if we search for answers in the sky and beneath our feet.

Patty asked me to do something similar: to look down and learn from the root systems of our trees.

We need our crip communities to flourish in the sustainability, trust, and care that the earth demonstrates around us. For Patty, and by extension for Sins Invalid, this is how we can achieve recurrent and loving bodymind change. We check in with one another. We resource share and communicate our boundaries. We share our harms, we discuss what is lacking, and we, as the performance project writes, articulate the movement forward.

―――――――――

"How much can we extend the invitation to get down?"

In thinking about how they can grow, create, and continue to learn, Sins Invalid invites the community to participate in their artist-activist and movement building work. Patty thinks through whether or not the project is staying true to Disability Justice by asking, "How much can we extend the invitation to get down?"[89] In other words, when Sins Invalid's Disability Justice–led practice urges that we should move without leaving anyone behind, who are we talking about? Who does *we* refer to? Who does *we* celebrate and who might it exclude? In their constant questioning of who might be missing, Sins Invalid has been able to respond to the community's concerns.

Some of this direction comes from the ways the performance project encourages mutual, collective knowledge gathering. For example, in preparing to write the second edition of *Skin, Tooth, and Bone,* Sins Invalid contacted their crip network to help them identify the gaps and pitfalls in the first edition. Respondents shared that the second edition needed to add a glossary of key terms and Disability Justice timelines as well as sections on audism, Deaf culture, and environmental illnesses. In their introduction, Sins Invalid also acknowledged that "We also tried to make our language more accessible and less academic. We have a long way to go in creating a disability justice primer that is actually accessible to people of all different cognitive styles and abilities."[90] Part of this cross-disability solidarity work for Sins Invalid returns to always remembering the yet-to-be labor and dreaming of Disability Justice; the main way to do this is by involving and requesting the community's wisdom.

There is so much love and humbleness embedded in Patty's questioning of *we* and this is part of what excites me about Sins Invalid and their Disability Justice–centered art-activism: we grow, heal, and learn in community and it is with our diverse communities that we are able to consider a multitude of knowledges. This is how, like the trees, we grow our brilliantly interconnected root systems.

———————

Sins Invalid's goal was never perfection. The goal continues to be an enactment of change, to continue community building, and to continue creating spaces that empower the resilience, beauty, and necessity of our bodyminds. Patty ended our conversation with this reminder about Sins Invalid's role: "It's about caring about people and loving people and wanting our conditions, both material and cultural conditions, to be grounded in dignity and generative sources of replenishment." My mind travels again and thinks of root systems, of mycelium, flocks of birds, and the trails and trails of ants in the backyard on this, the hottest day of the summer. The goal is interconnectivity and growth, the flourishing that is sometimes hard won, but always planted in love.

CHAPTER 4

Storytelling as Activism, as Crip-Centric Strategy

We, the disabled, the chronically ill, and the Mad carry within us archives. We are intergenerational memory banks filled with the labor, organizing, and artmaking of our radical disabled, queer of color contemporaries, elders, and ancestors. We carry stories of resilience and survival, stories of growth and trauma. In sharing our crip stories, we unearth legacies of colonialism and nondisabled supremacy. We, dear reader, craft ourselves new routes to follow.

Writer and professor Arthur W. Frank explores how stories refamiliarize and reroute our bodyminds, especially if we are disabled or chronically ill.[91] He writes that "the personal issue of telling stories about [disability and] illness is to give voice to the body, so that the changed body can become once again familiar in these stories.... The body is often alienated, literally 'made strange,' as it is told in stories that are instigated by the need to make it familiar."[92] We tell our stories as a way to speak for our bodyminds. With these stories we create new routes and new maps back to ourselves. Because so many of us often do not speak in our own voices and are instead, spoken for, disabled storytelling is a radical act. Sometimes, medical professionals deny our bodymind knowledges, patronizing and dismissing us. Sometimes, the voices of our doctors, our therapists, our social workers, our family members, and the medical industrial complex overwhelm us and become our voices until we are made unfamiliar, or to use Arthur's language, made strange, even to ourselves.

Crip-centric liberated zones can serve as places where we become recognizable to ourselves, again; they can become places that empower us with a new map, with a new route. As a crip-centric liberated zone, Sins Invalid's use of storytelling as activism is a way for us to return to our abundant disabled, queer of color splendor. There is power in the act of naming bodymind experiences just as there is power in witnessing another's story and perhaps finding homecoming in them. The disabled, queer of color bodymind stories in this chapter not only give voice to experiences silenced by ableism and historical lineages of oppression, but they also serve as crip, queer, decolonial love maps for the community. Here, we become more than Otherness, deviance, and damage. Here we become lifeblood.

"Before I can even tell you a story, you need to really love and praise yourself."

Before we can enter ourselves in stories, before we can become familiar to ourselves once again and embark upon a new route, we first need to learn how to love our bodyminds. Alice Wong communicates this best when she writes, "There is power in storytelling. Before I can even tell you a story, you need to really love and praise yourself. You need to say that 'I do have a story, that I do matter.'"[93] Inhabiting our bodymind stories requires reflection. It requires the realization that our stories are valid and valuable, that they deserve to be told, and that they carry so much more than our forced, ableist narratives of shame. It is a decolonizing act to lean into this reality and to remember ourselves *past*: *past* the history of colonization and extracted economies, *past* eugenics, the limitations of the medical industrial complex, and *past* ableism's mandates. To use storytelling as a way to move *past* into a transformed disabled, queer of color future where all our bodyminds matter is Disability Justice and its love work.

For Sins Invalid, the use of storytelling moves us closer toward ourselves; it moves us closer toward connection-building with our communities. Sammie Ablaza Wills (they/them), Director of APIENC (Asian Pacific Islander Equality–Northern California), describes this best when they talk about how reclamation journeys need care and slowness. I heard Sammie speak during a webinar hosted by Movement Generation's Course Correction series in July 2020.[94] The goal of the webinar was to transport us to the future, to the year 2050, a time when we have arrived at liberation for the people. In their talk, Sammie imagined a place where "we are relearning each other as the plants do, with patience and care." As they spoke, I imagined plants growing, tendrils bending and folding into one another. I imagined the earth reminding us how to move ourselves back to a place of tenderness. This is the work of cripped storytelling: in slowness and care, we learn to love ourselves outside of oppressive frameworks. We love ourselves enough to create crip-centric liberated zones.

———————

Telling our bodymind stories is a crip strategy for liberation and it begins with the telling of what Arthur W. Frank calls "embodied stories."[95] Embodied stories are the stories that disabled folks share about their bodyminds, through their bodyminds. It is an empowered act of reclamation to reach into ourselves for our stories in search of what might be lost. When I asked Patty about why Sins Invalid used storytelling as a method of crip thriving, she/they told me that embracing and telling one's own story heals us.[96] Healing our bodyminds through storytelling reroutes us back to ourselves: our languages, our stories, and our experiences, all told in our own voices as we manifest them. Storytelling creates a profound reverberation that reaches outward and welcomes disabled and nondisabled folks alike to reexplore what disability means outside of the framings of ableism, sanism, audism, and all of the systems of discrimination that marginalize and oppress the extraordinary diversity of our disability community.

When I think about how storytelling helps us unlearn the regressive bodymind lessons we have been taught, I think about crip poet Maria Palacios. Maria is a Texas-based Latina, writer-activist, and a regular on the Sins Invalid stage. In her 2009 spoken word performance "Testimony," she uses storytelling to make her body familiar to herself. On stage, she sits in her wheelchair facing a mirror that is draped with a black shawl. Haloed in a pink light, Maria begins by speaking to the mirror: "I used to hate my body, cringe at the thought of a mirror, deformities staring at me. *Pobricita, poor little thing. Shhh, don't look, don't ask.* That's when I was cripple girl in a Barbie world. *Shhh, don't talk, she'll never walk, she'll never know love.* The mirror used to say that, and I used

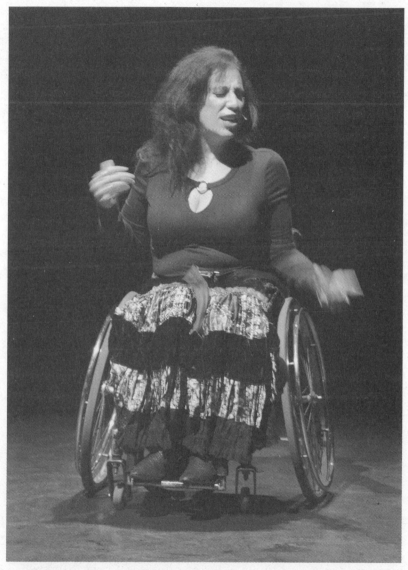

Maria Palacios in "Testimony", 2008. *Sins Invalid Annual Performance*, Brava Theater. Photo by Richard Downing, courtesy of Sins Invalid.

to believe it." "Testimony" begins with ableist declarations about Maria's body: her disability was something to tolerate and pity; it was wound and damage.[97] The myth that beauty means nondisability and whiteness, that only beautiful bodies are worthy of love, colonized Maria. She faces the audience, her voice pleading, pained, and distraught at these memories. She evokes Barbie and Cinderella in the performance, calling forward these mythic, symbolic ideals of Eurocentric, nondisabled beauty. They are the ghosts and specters that haunt and shame her.

In many ways, this performance is a journey, a rerouting toward self-love and tenderness. Maria doesn't reclaim her bodymind story until she moves through her own internalized ableism. She must first excavate her past reflection and her feelings of shame before she can realize, as Alice urges, that her story matters. For Maria, creating a new map and moving past means confrontation. It means agitating and unlearning past narratives that swallow whole and erase her own crip magic. Moving past means reclaiming her bodymind through storytelling.

When Maria engages in this shift, her voice and her body language change. She becomes certain and cradles herself with her arms: "My present testimony is a manifesto of self-love, reconciliation between mirror and soul." Storytelling here for Maria becomes liberatory. In altering her bodymind story, Maria also alters her sense of self. In her exploration of body image and body positivity, Sonya Renee Taylor writes, "For so many of us, *sorry* has become how we translate the word *body*."[98] I extend this conflation to disability, to the taught impulse that we must always apologize for our disabled, chronically ill, Mad body-minds, that we must always provide an answer to the question, *what happened to you?* By the end of the performance, through storytelling,

Maria no longer sees herself as an apology or deformity. Rather, she becomes a radical manifestation of cripped self-love.

_____

"Storytelling is cultural activism."

When Leroy F. Moore Jr. and I spoke in 2016 about the importance of storytelling, especially for the artists that perform with Sins Invalid, he emphasized that they are putting voice and movement to the narratives that are difficult but most necessary to hear. He said that Sins Invalid becomes "the place where we can finally tell our stories as brown crips, as queer crips. [It's where we can] tell the story of our ancestors. This sto rytelling is cultural activism. Many of these stories are hard to swallow but they need to be swallowed. I think some people see storytelling as, *oh, it's so pretty and it's really a good story*, but there are also hard stories that shape our foundation, and they need to be heard."[99] Storytelling as activism becomes remembrance, becomes genealogy. Sometimes the stories we tell about our bodyminds are the ones full of grit and sweat. They are the painful stories, the *I have never said this out loud* stories, the *this is the most vulnerable I have ever been* stories. Because stories can uncover and give voice to those who are unseen, marginalized, and forgotten, Leroy positions storytelling as an activist act.

In this conversation of activist storytelling, I need to evoke Chicana lesbian feminist Gloria Anzaldúa and her rebellious, moving, jerking, "wild tongue."[100] In her book *Borderlands/La Frontera*, she reflects on her tongue's active resistance while at the dentist: "My tongue keeps pushing out the wads of cotton, pushing back the drills, the long nee-dles. 'I've never seen anything as strong or as stubborn,' he says. And I think, how do you tame a wild tongue, train it to be quiet, how do you bridle and saddle it? How do you make it lie down?"[101] As I reread this passage from a place informed by disabled, queer of color liberation, I think about Gloria's wild tongue as a metaphor: we, the disabled, queer of color many have always existed. We are the tongue. We are persistent in being heard. We exist, willful, even when our own communities render us invisible and silent, even when our stories remain untold. The wild tongue represents our endurance and creates new routes and new ways of thriving. This lesson of fortitude for Sins Invalid arrives when we gather and tell our stories. Storytelling in this way becomes our vulnerable tenacity to continue, despite.

Gloria declares herself with her tongue. She writes that as a queer Chicana[102] she "will no longer be made to feel ashamed of existing. I will have my voice ... I will overcome the tradition of silence."[103] From this place, storytelling becomes an embodiment of decolonized and cripped self-love; it becomes the act of moving past: moving past shame and silence, past oppressions that censor us, and even past our own internalizations of disempowerment. In moving past, we are able to search out and declare our authentic selves in all our deliberate relentlessness. It is the realization that although medicine always tells stories about our bodyminds, cripping storytelling can help us retell our stories so that we are no longer damage, defect, or shame. Here, we become our own storytellers.

In the fifth episode of *Crip Bits*, the bimonthly Facebook series organized by Patty and the Sins Invalid community, Patty spoke about the medical industrial complex's propensity for silencing disabled, queer of color bodyminds. Not only do medical narratives colonize us with their ableist, racist, and cis-heteropatriarchal frameworks, but they also exercise ownership over us, our bodyminds, and our stories.[104]

In sharing bodymind stories from this marginal place, Sins Invalid invests in and prioritizes bodymind reclamation; they challenge the forced, structural silences that reduce us to stereotype by giving disabled, queer of color artists a platform to be heard. This, returning to Leroy's argument, is what it means to position storytelling as activism, to use storytelling as a way to challenge sedimented thought and to bring about social change. This type of cultural activism, as Patty shared on *Crip Bits*, happens when we are not "dismissed" or "scripted over ... in nonconsensual ways."[105] The coming chapters in this book will continue to explore specific Sins Invalid performances, community events, and workshops to demonstrate how this art-activist storytelling occurs, what it looks like, and how it creates sacred space for disabled, queer of color community to witness themselves as radiant and whole.

———

"Open up. Make room. Let the circle grow."

In her 2011 performance for Sins Invalid, writer, artist, and activist Aurora Levins Morales wrote and performed a poem set to movement. As a collaboration between Aurora; Patty; and African and Indigenous, Deaf, two-spirit dancer Antoine Hunter (he/him), "Listen, Speak" serves as one of the many examples of what activist storytelling means, how it liberates, and how it helps us remember the ancestors who have always existed. Wearing white shorts and painted in a chalky white, Antoine stagger-walks through the audience toward the stage. His arms bow outward as if he is holding something heavy; we soon learn that this is the weight of history; this is the weight of bodies owned, sold, and dehumanized.

Aurora's voice booms overhead: "Open up. Make room. Let the circle grow. From the shadows steps a man from Tuskegee, syphilis raging untreated through his veins, gone blind, lame, and speechless while white doctors took notes, but here he speaks with a voice like a drum." Antoine holds up a white scarf against the light as Aurora speaks. The stage is dark, but the scarf catches the light; a projector displays images of chain link fences and hands on the fabric. He covers his face as he spins; he holds his body stiff, and his movement is repetitive. It isn't until the end of the piece that Antoine's limbs become fluid, his feet planted securely, while his arms gesture upward. Again, we hear Aurora: "We unwrap our tongues, we bind our stories, we choose to be naked, we show our markings, we lick our fingers, we stroke our bellies, we laugh at midnight, we change the ending, we begin, and begin again." Her words tell the story of scientific racism and enslavement. It is a history of the Tuskegee Experiments, the medical exploitation and oppression of over six hundred Black men in the United States. This performance calls us to remember.

In many ways, "Listen, Speak" serves as knowledge sharing. It is a retelling of poor, Black, disabled, and chronically ill bodyminds. It is a reminder that, as Aurora says in the beginning of her piece, "Our history is in our bodies." We cannot journey toward collective liberation without reclaiming our bodymind histories, voices, and stories. Storytelling in this way is cyclical. It results in the storyteller bearing witness to themselves while also inviting others to access that same awareness and vulnerability. It is a place where we can gather together to create connection and kinship, where disabled, queer of color bodyminds can engage in the implicit change-making that is storytelling.[106]

"The story becomes a way of remaking the world."

In addition to its activist goals, storytelling by disabled, queer of color bodyminds also creates community. Just as it creates homecoming, it also centers what writer and activist Kayhan Irani names a story's potential to identify "obstacles to freedom, to health, to safety, and to dignity."[107] When we tell the bodymind stories we have been told to keep hidden, when we use storytelling to challenge the oppressions that threaten to swallow us whole, we are, as Kayhan says, naming what forcibly distances us from dignity. With our telling, we stake claim to our bodyminds. Our stories become the ways in which we demand our collective freedom and safety, the ways in which we remind the world that we are deserving.

Storytelling by disabled, queer of color bodyminds embraces Disability Justice and its principle of collective liberation. It prioritizes communities whose voices have been forcibly restrained. It creates a platform where majoritarian stories, stories that are told from places of power and privilege, are troubled, and where assumptions of what a "normal" bodymind looks like are severed at their core.[108] In their seminal work exploring counter-storytelling, education scholars Daniel G. Solórzano and Tara J. Yosso explore how majoritarian stories rely on the assumption that some identities are "good" while others are "bad": "Morally, the silence within which assumptions are made about good versus bad describes people of color and working-class people as less intelligent and irresponsible while depicting White middle-class and upper-class people as just the opposite."[109] Beyond race and class, majoritarian stories have also taught us that nondisability and heterosexuality are good, while disability and queerness are inherently bad.

The disabled, queer of color bodyminds that refuse this oppressive narrative engage in counter-storytelling, an activist narrative exercise that resists assimilation.[110] Counter-storytelling is Gloria's wild tongue, jolting and refusing shame; it is the wild tongue's rebel voice. Oppressed communities reach into their pasts, their presents, and their futures to tell stories of their bodyminds as survival and reclamation, as a way to, as Kayhan reminds us, "remake the world."[111] Remaking the world here becomes an expression of collective liberation, an urging that we craft ways of moving together so that no one is left behind.[112] If Disability Justice as a framework and practice upholds the legacies of our disabled, queer of color ancestors, then storytelling for Sins Invalid is one way to get us there. To position disabled queer of color stories as liberatory counter-stories teaches us that adopting stigma is more than toxic; it eradicates.

Stories also move us to recall the lives of those who were "never meant to survive," as Audre Lorde writes in her 1978 poem "A Litany for Survival": "For those of us who live at the shoreline / … For those of us / who were imprinted with fear / like a faint line on our foreheads / … For all of us this instead and this triumph / We were never meant to survive." Most poignantly, counter-storytelling helps our bodyminds resist erasure so that they can be brought back and made discernable once again. Sins Invalid employs storytelling as strategy, as declaration: we are here despite intergenerational trauma, despite the medical industrial complex, despite all in this world that wants to eradicate us. Our stories are our proof.

———————

Cara Page's opening for Sins Invalid's 2009 evening of performance art demonstrates liberatory counter-storytelling at its finest. As the MC for the evening, Cara stands on stage against a black backdrop. She wears a black corset and skirt, and her eyelashes extend well past her cheeks. Cara begins by opening Sins Invalid to us as an intentional space of counter-storytelling: "Welcome to our queendom, kingdom, queer-dom, multibodied universe. I will be your mistress of dreams, creating new divinations for our bodies and through our souls. Tonight, we will be new maps of celestial beings, new constellations setting course for our collective bodies and shapes to create what freedom and love can look like, feel like, taste like, without any perfect body, any perfect shape or form. Without assuming any single way of thinking or desire. There is no right or wrong body of a conscious revolutionary mind." Cara's language here evokes the welcoming of diverse genders, sexualities, and bodyminds. Her centering of these communities is, in and of itself, a revolutionary practice of counter-storytelling that mobilizes narrative as a tool for "remaking of the world." Cara's use of the word "maps" also returns me to the beginning of this chapter and the argument that our bodymind stories create new destinations and pathways for our dis-abled, queer of color bodyminds. We, as Cara reminds us, can follow these maps to our collective thriving.

In reflecting on the origins of the *Disability Visibility Project*, Alice Wong says that the project most importantly "was giving all of us a way to tell our own stories, in our own words, without waiting around for

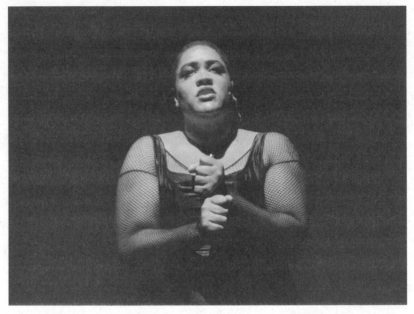

MC Cara Page, 2008. *Sins Invalid Annual Performance*, Brava Theater. Photo by Richard Downing, courtesy of Sins Invalid.

a historian to find us significant."[113] Sins Invalid's performance community similarly knows that disabled, queer of color presence, impact, and worth should not be contingent on formalized recognition. We design and elevate our own cripped, queered, decolonial paths to ensure that we, in justice, flourish. Cara moves us toward this solution when she offers that "Tonight we will be new maps of celestial beings, new constellations setting course for our collective bodies and shapes to create what freedom and love can look like." Guided by an intrinsic and furious refusal to wait, Sins Invalid writes us free by amplifying the bodymind stories we carry within us.

Patty shared with me that the performance project's focus on storytelling "allows people to experience a liberation of self in the audience. It's a palpable feeling of liberation and emotional connecting. To me this is what liberation can look like. We can create self-love and respect for each other."[14] Whether their stories are expressed through writing or movement workshops or through their evenings of multidisciplinary art, Sins Invalid engages with storytelling to help us reroute our way back to our bodyminds in revolutionary love. In bearing witness to disabled, queer of color stories, we are reminded of the worth and value of our histories, our experiences, and our bodyminds. For some of us, it is the first time we are given refuge, the first time we feel empowered in the untold, the first time we become aware of our potential to remake and confront this ableist, racist, cis-heteropatriarchal world. Storytelling from this crip, queer of color perspective is how we move past, and it is how we learn to stay.

CHAPTER 5

Artmaking as Evidence

Since their birthing, Sins Invalid engages with multidisciplinary artmaking to embolden and sustain crip-centric liberated zones. Art made by disabled, queer of color community becomes sustenance and strategy for crip-centric resilience. Similar to storytelling, artmaking gives us a voice and a language with which to love our bodyminds in the face of intersecting oppressions. This type of politicized artmaking moves disability past shame and toward pride and liberation. Here, liberation becomes modern dance choreographed by Deaf dancers. Liberation becomes a crip striptease performed on a wheelchair. It becomes an unlearning of a past of emotional abuses through poetry. Liberation becomes challenge, transformation, and potential.

Patty and Leroy have worked to ensure that Sins Invalid recognizes, revises, and centers the identities of the disabled, queer of color communities it supports. They knew that they wanted to "address the disconnect between what we know to be true about our beauty and what the world seems to believe—that we are 'less than,' undesirable and pitiable."[115] As artist-activists who are familiar with the transformative ways art becomes exercise and lifeline, Patty and Leroy wanted to support artmaking that names and expresses our bodyminds on our own terms. As fertile home, the performance project became the place where disabled, queer of color creators could explore and decolonize their bodymind narratives with the intent of redefining themselves through art. This is what the connecting of art and activism does: it mobilizes and creates profound social change. It gifts us with the ability to ignite a self and communal recognition that reroutes us back to our luscious, disabled, queer of color selves.

Building Disabled, Queer of Color Art-Activism

As a performance project, Sins Invalid engages in both multidisciplinary art creation as well as their Disability Justice activism; their intersection of art-activism answers visual artist and activist Kirsten Dufour's call, "What can art do?"[116] Extending this, the performance project asks us to consider, to reimagine, and to remake what disabled, queer of color bodyminds can do and what transformations they can create. How can "art as activism"[117] made by Sins Invalid expand the lessons we have been taught about disability?

"Art as activism" is a concept from English professor Deborah Barndt's book *Wild Fire: Art as Activism*. In unpacking the connections between these two, she writes, "Whether the modes of expression are verbal or non-verbal, artmaking that ignites people's creativity, recovers repressed histories, builds community and strengthens social movements is in itself a holistic form of action."[118] Engaging in art creation informed by Disability Justice develops for us language for social change, visibility, and remembering. Sins Invalid's art-activism reclaims a "political imagination"[119] that is at once disabled, queer, and of color.

Patty engages with the phrase "political imagination" in an interview with Leroy by CulturalOrganizing dot org. After Leroy shares that for Sins Invalid there is no separation between activism and art movements, Patty responds:

> Sometimes people think of cultural activism as the soft front of a move-ment, but we think that's not accurate. I firmly believe that capitalism is winning because it has stolen the political imagination. We need to take that political imagination back. Obviously, we have to engage in condi-tions, we have to address oppression, but that's not the end of our vision. As cultural workers it's our responsibility to hold a broader vision of what it means to be a woman of color, what it means to be a person with a disability, what it means to be a man who has cerebral palsy. Our vision has to be greater than what we can access from dominant culture.[120]

To regain our political imagination requires fierce dreaming and radical self-love. It requires, to return to Sara Ahmed, a willful resistance to all the ways we have been taught to view our disabled, queer of color bodyminds. For Patty, this defiant and daring practice has far-reaching implications for change-making. Sins Invalid invites us to activate our political imaginations; they invite us to frame our bodyminds as beauti-ful and worthy, as emboldened with deep, sustainable, interdependent lessons.

I want to pause here on sustainability as a cripped out tactic for thriv-ing in an ableist world, as it is one of the central organizing principles for both Sins Invalid and Disability Justice. As the sixth principle of

Disability Justice, sustainability advocates that "we learn to pace our-selves, individually and collectively, to be sustained long-term. We value the teaching of our bodies and experiences and use them as a critical guide and reference point to help us move away from urgency."[121] Our bodyminds do not merely sustain us. They teach us. They are language and possibility, and this principle of Disability Justice asks that we listen to them—in all the diverse ways we engage in listening. Arising from the exhaustion and burnout culture of capitalism and the exhaustion that organizers and activists also experience when a movement does not consider the bodymind, sustainability reminds us that it is necessary to slow down, look inward, and honestly assess what our bodyminds can and cannot do. There is no judgement here. Power exists in both doing *and* in not doing, in saying, *no, not today*. Perhaps most powerfully, this principle expands our collective political imagination around time and productivity.[122]

Direct outgrowths of sustainability include crip time, what Mad Studies scholar and professor Margaret Price calls a "flexible approach to normative time frames."[123] Crip time "bend[s] the clock to meet dis-abled bodies and minds."[124] It is a breaking of time[125] that opens in its place slowness and consideration so that our disabled bodyminds can exist as they are and as they need to.[126] For Sins Invalid, sustainability in movement organizing and artmaking is realizing that it is more import-ant to postpone a scheduled performance when staff and performers get sick and do not have the capacity to work than it is to push on as ableism and capitalism would have us do. Crip time and sustainability honor *need*. Sustainability, in particular, tells us that there is no shame in mov-ing slow, in making sure that we are fed and rested before we contribute to the revolution. It is an enactment of crip love to ask of ourselves and one another, *what is your capacity? What does your bodymind need?*

———————

Embracing art as activism offers us possibilities. With their engagement of art as an expression of Disability Justice, Sins Invalid's performances give us interventions for a political strategy that uplifts disabled, queer of color community. Their application of art as Disability Justice activism provokes and renders messy the belief that, returning to their mission statement, only nondisabled bodyminds are sexy and beautiful. Through their art-activism we enter Sins Invalid's cripped imaginations.

As a direct outgrowth of their art-activist practice, the performance project also produces community-based cultural programming. By the end of 2008, three years after they began, their programming had reached nearly two thousand people throughout the United States. These free, accessible, crip-centric community workshops and Disability Justice trainings envisioned the disabled as agentic, as emboldened with the power for tender and fierce change-making: for example, performer Rodney Bell led a movement-based workshop named "Moving in Grace"; poet Maria Palacios and Leroy led "Tongue Rhythm," a poetry workshop; and community activist Noemi Sohn and Patty led "Come as You Are," a workshop that explored the erotic powers of writing. As expressions of Sins Invalid's mission statement, these workshops provide educational, crip-centric opportunities for healing in the face of the many institutions that can restrict and harm us.

Art-activism, whether on stage as performances or within the community as workshops, began for Sins Invalid with the goal of solidarity, of cripping, queering, and decolonizing mainstream nondisabled representations of how a disabled, queer of color bodymind must dance, move, create, and navigate this world. This work historically comes from the politicized tradition of the mainstream Disability Rights Movement and the 1970s disability arts movement.[127] Disability Studies scholar Allan Sutherland names the reciprocal relationship between disability politics and the disability arts movement this way: "I don't think disability arts would have been possible without disability politics coming first ... Our art draws upon our politics, but it also feeds back into it."[128] To create from this activist place results in self-discovery and love. There is a remaking of the world here, too. Art becomes another medium through which disabled, queer of color bodyminds can generate new, liberatory pathways on which to travel.

"We must leave evidence, evidence that we were here, that we existed ..."

Leaving Evidence is the name of Disability Justice and Transformative Justice activist Mia Mingus's blog. I reference the title and goal of her blog here as a strategy and larger metaphor, as a way for us to understand the art-activist effects of Sins Invalid's performances. It is a profound and transformative act to leave evidence that we lived, that we struggled, and that we thrived. Sometimes, we are so erased by the intersecting oppressions that regulate our bodyminds that all we can do to remember that we exist and that we deserve to exist is to leave evidence, to leave proof that we were here. To resist this erasure, we offer bodymind maps of endurance; we offer our stories, our faces, and our histories so that we too can become tangible.

In an interview with Alice Wong, Mia unpacks the importance of leaving evidence. She shares that "we must leave evidence, evidence that we were here, that we existed, that we survived and loved and ate. Evidence of the wholeness we never felt. An immense sense of fullness we gave each other. Evidence of who we were, and who we thought we were, who we never should have been. Evidence of each other, and there are other ways to live past survival, past isolation."[129] Leaving evidence signals our arrival. It is a beacon, a lighthouse bringing our disabled, queer of color communities home. For Mia, leaving evidence means that we acknowledge the good and the difficult parts of being disabled.[130] It is a vulnerable act to leave behind the honest, messy, and painful stories about our bodyminds. It is the admittance that our disabled lives are complex and comprised of pride and struggle, that we deserve to exist surrounded by community, just as we are. When we recognize that we deserve to exist, we become the storytellers of our own lives; we become wild tongues, speak-spitting evidence.

Sins Invalid's performances leave us evidence that our disabled bodyminds are worthy, sexy, whole, and beautiful; our queerness, our trans and gender nonconformity, our bodyminds of color, all beautiful, all radiant, all necessary in this world. This politic grounds itself in the Disability Justice principle of collective liberation, the call that we "leave no bodymind behind"[131] as we imagine our futures. The performance project's work leaves evidence so that others in search of community and homecoming can find their way. They offer us proof that we not only exist, but that we deserve to exist. This is, after all, what evidence can become: proof of our bodyminds, proof of our necessity and relevance, proof that a new crip culture of collective liberation exists. This is Sins Invalid's vision: to use artmaking and performance work to shift the toxic paradigms that eradicate so many of us and make us unknown even to ourselves.

_____

"It was very painful to argue that we have a right to exist."

Patty and Leroy are intimately familiar with the history of crip erasure. As a wheelchair user, Patty experienced crip erasure each time she/ they were approached by strangers who wanted to pray over her/them and banish her/their body's "curse." Crip erasure is Leroy being told, as he waited for a bus, "You useless cripple, you go home!"[132] Regardless of context or location, crip erasure always eradicates. It reinstates the medical model of disability, reducing our disabled, chronically ill, Mad bodyminds to defect, deviance, and pathology. Crip erasure moves us far away from ourselves, our hearts, and our rebel spirits. It isolates us from ourselves and our history, from our communities and from the power of disabled, queer of color kinship. In its wake we fail to remember that we are beauty, that we are empowered, and that we, as Sins Invalid reminds, are "an essential part of humanity."[133] Crip erasure makes us forget that we are evidence, and most powerfully, that we can leave evidence.

_____

These moments of erasure and forgetting are always around us. When I first began this project in 2016, two moments in particular sedimented me in the trauma that is crip erasure and reminded me of why we need Sins Invalid's art-activism and Disability Justice resistance. The first moment took place on July 26, 2016, in Sagamihara, Kanagawa

Prefecture, Japan. Nineteen disabled residents nine men and ten women—were murdered at the Tsukui Yamayuri-en residential care facility. Satoshi Uematsu, a former employee, committed the murders. In an interview with Japanese newspaper *The Mainichi,* he said that he murdered the residents "for the sake of society," that the disabled have "no point in living," that they "only create unhappiness."[134] Satoshi believed in eugenics and used it to justify his violence.[135] Eugenics, whether it is sterilizing or euthanizing disabled folks, serves as legalized and tangible crip erasure. It is a traumatic elimination that reinforces nondisabled supremacy's mandate that disabilities and the disabled community must be eliminated.

There are two key aspects of this story that replicate nondisabled supremacy's repeated message that disabled bodyminds are disposable and must remain invisible. When these murders first occurred, US and world news coverage was minimal. They did not increase until Satoshi's court case began, and they peaked when he was sentenced in March 2020.[136] Nondisabled supremacy teaches us over and over again that not everyone's story matters, that not everyone's bodymind experience matters. This realization was compounded for me when I read that the families of the murdered residents refused to release their names due to the stigma of disability. Shame erases evidence; in this case, shame erases crip lives. There was a moment of resistance to crip erasure, however, during Satoshi's sentencing in the spring of 2020. One family decided to share their daughter's name and story and, in doing so, they left evidence: "Her name was Miho. I want that public as proof that she existed. I want people to know who she was."[137] Leaving evidence in this way confronts crip erasure and reframes disabled bodyminds as meaningful, as *always* meaningful.

The second moment of crip erasure was the story of fourteen-year-old Jerika Bolen. Jerika lived in Appleton, Wisconsin. She was a Black, disabled, and queer teen who was preparing to remove her ventilator and die at the end of August 2016. Diagnosed with spinal muscular atrophy type 2, Jerika's story sparked debates and reflections around autonomy, agency, and, ultimately, the need for crip community. In a Facebook post, Patty shared that she/they intimately understood Bolen, her life experiences, and her pain: "Don't think I fault Jerika at all—she is 14 yrs [sic] old and growing up within the uninterrupted ableism of Appleton, Wisconsin, within its barely interrupted white supremacy and misogynoir. She is 14 and deserving of guidance, of crip love, of black and brown women's crip centered reflections of her incalculable worth, of her gifts that only she can bring into the world." Patty frames crip community as guide, as doula.[138] Crip community creates space for our injured spirits, teaches us, and listens. Crip community brings us home. Disabled, queer of color community, in particular, can nourish and embrace intersectional living, all of its excitement and its fertile messiness. According to Patty and many folks in the Disability Justice community, Jerika's story might have been different if she were surrounded by the lessons of disabled, queer of color community, lessons of how to unsettle all that is privileged as normal, how to live in collective access, and how to embody sexy crip living; her story might have been different if she had seen evidence.

Prom was a key part of Jerika's story, what news outlets called "her last dance." On Friday, July 22, 2016, friends, family, and strangers gathered in the Grand Meridian ballroom in Appleton. They wore dresses, ate, and danced. Before arriving at the ballroom, Jerika and her friends and family were led into town by a motorcade. Appleton's Police Chief

Todd Thomas told a reporter, "We're just blessed to help out … It's an honor for us, and what an amazing young lady. She makes you appreciate what you have. She makes you think about using your time wisely. She's making an impact."[139] Reading this was a gut-punch. Jerika was meant to inspire the nondisabled to live life fully and without reservation. She was what disability activist Stella Young aptly defines as "inspiration porn." By objectifying her as inspirational, Jerika's only purpose was to galvanize the living, something she continues to do even after her death on September 22, 2016. Objectifying her story erases her resilience, her Blackness, and her queerness. Objectifying her story erases Jerika's crip future.

––––––––––

In reflecting on eugenics and the ways the medical industrial complex, particularly reproductive technologies, view disability as a defect, Patty says that perhaps one of the most agonizing parts of crip erasure is the labor of having to constantly prove your worth and that you deserve to live. For Sins Invalid, disabled, queer of color storytelling and artmaking serve as politicized tools for crip survival and crip recognition. They give audience members and performers an embodied language for fighting disabled, queer of color erasure; they provide us with a map to move closer and closer toward the Disability Justice framing that "All bodies and minds are unique and essential. All bodies are whole. All bodies have strengths and needs that must be met. We are powerful not despite the complexities of our bodies, but because of them. We move together with no body left behind."[140] Much of Sins Invalid's art-activism begins here, by focusing on the ways we can combat the violence and oppression of crip erasure and learn how to reroute ourselves toward what feminist studies and disability studies scholar Alison Kafer calls a "collective reimagining" of what disability means and what it can do.[141]

During Sins Invalid's 2009 performance, UK-based disabled actor, writer, and performance artist Mat Fraser highlights the struggle of proving our worth, the struggle of proving that we are deserving. His piece, "No Retreat, No Surrender," forces us to confront the effects of ableism and the embodied and enminded[142] trauma of crip erasure. As the piece begins, the visual marker of Mat's shortened arms—his mother was prescribed Thalidomide when he was in utero—are contrasted against his kicking, swinging legs, and their pushing defiance. The lighting on stage is purple. As Mat moves, the theater is overwhelmed with the sound of ableist attacks; the conversations overlap loudly. He plants his legs and begins kickboxing an invisible attacker who booms overhead, "You are very, very brave. You are my hero of the day. It's so good for my kids to have you as a disabled friend." So many of us in the disability community have been told that we are courageous and heroic simply because we are disabled and alive. I return to Jerika's story here, to the symbol of inspiration and bravery into which nondisabled supremacy coercively fashioned her. Mat's body resists this narrative and with determination, he attacks.

As these voices continue, they become more caustic, and they push Mat off his feet. He falls to the floor as the assaults overhead continue: "I'm sorry you are going to have to sit at another seat ... Did your mother feel guilty? ... Do you need help making love? You can work at the storeroom but not at the register ... Reproduction is a mistake. Creating another deformity is a disaster ... Looking at your arms makes me feel sick. I would never fuck a cripple." Just as quickly as Mat gets up, he falls down. The invisible attacker punches his face and his head jolts

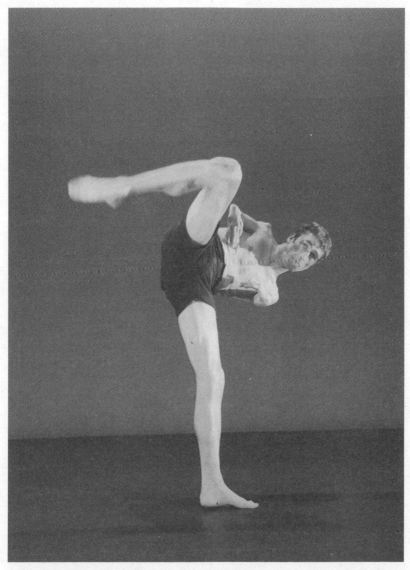

Mat Fraser in "No Retreat, No Surrender", 2009. *Sins Invalid Annual Performance*, Brava Theater. Photo by Richard Downing, courtesy of Sins Invalid.

back. These phrases patronize and dismember. Blood begins to pour from his mouth as his body lifts up only to fall back down again. By the end of the performance, Mat's limp body is dragged off stage.

This performance communicates, perhaps better than any dictation of history or discussion of ableism, that the fight is not yet over. Our disabled bodyminds still encounter daily oppressions and we still actively need to imagine a crip future where we matter, where we thrive beyond the rhetorics of inspiration and tokenism. Mat's performance invites us to acknowledge the persistence of the tangible lived realities of nondisabled supremacy so that we, in our reimaginings and reroutings, can recognize ourselves as valuable, whole, and as truly transformational crip beings.

_____

"Finding beauty in that which we have been told is abject and disposable has profound implications."

The revision of the disabled bodymind as sexy, desiring, and beautiful is a central theme and foundational performance element for Sins Invalid; it serves as an integral part of disabled, queer of color recognition. Within their crip-centric liberated zones, we can define beauty as expansive and rhythmic. Its standards can shift, stretching to include and honor all our bodyminds. In this place, we can reimagine beauty outside of capitalism, outside of nondisability, white supremacy, and cis-heteropatriarchy. We can, instead, enter into a flirtatious, luscious dreamscape where we combat crip erasure by offering a new crip-centric definition of beauty. To acknowledge disabled bodyminds as sexy, as something other than damage or disgust, foregrounds beauty as action, as a cripped lexicon that inherently centers disabled, queer of color bodyminds.

Perhaps the most powerful entry point of crip beauty is the way it fractures ableism's assumption that beauty is only reserved for the non-disabled. During a discussion with Sins Invalid members and Disability Justice and Trans Liberation activists, gender nonconforming perfor-mance artist and writer Alok Vaid-Menon (they/them) advocates that we must remember that beauty is more than the superficial: "We are taught to desire the very things that destroy us, and we are taught to fear the very things that have the potential to set us free. Finding beauty in that which we have been told is abject or disposable has profound impli-cations."[143] Performing disabled, queer of color frameworks of beauty teaches us that our bodyminds are extraordinary, rather than abject and disposable. Beauty here becomes the limp, becomes burned glossy skin, and abundant drool. Beauty becomes Mad minds rapid loving and stim-ming hands. It is the survival magic of all our bodyminds doing beauty by blurring boundaries.

Since we are so often taught that disabled bodyminds are child-like and desexual, Sins Invalid ensures that sexuality and eroticism are also woven into each evening of performance art. Although each performance has a unique theme, sexuality and beauty are constants. Repetition, here, becomes strategy; it becomes a way to leave evidence that disabled folks are, as Patty says, "hot—super hot in fact! It's super sexy to see people engaged with their lives, doin' themselves."[144]

Crip beauty is Lateef McLeod, a Black disabled poet and activist, walk-ing on stage during Sins Invalid's 2016 performance. Lateef wears a

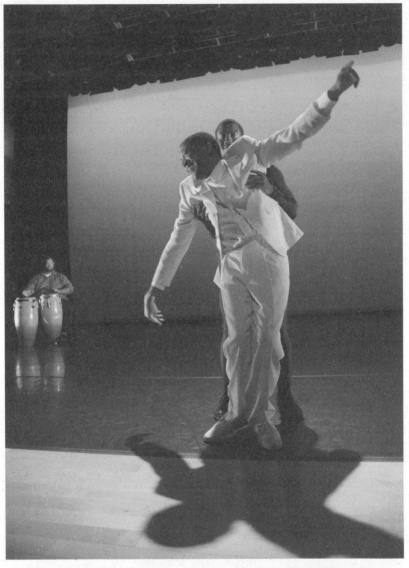

Lateef McLeod, 2016. *Birthing, Dying, Becoming Crip Wisdom*, ODC Theater. Photo by Richard Downing, courtesy of Sins Invalid.

white suit, walks rigidly, and is supported by a man who stands behind him. As he points, smiles, and shifts his body weight, a narrator reads his poem: "My children, you are beautifully and wonderfully made ... Don't be fooled ... you were not a mistake. I molded and crafted your bodies as masterpieces." We are not disposable. Our disabilities do not render us abject mistakes. We are, as Lateef says, masterpieces. This is crip beauty, the visibility of a disabled bodymind of color who exists outside the myth of error, just exactly as he should.

Crip beauty is a film montage that played during the same 2016 show. We are presented with close-ups of faces. In this silent and slow montage, we are asked to bear witness to people whose faces have been burned or scarred. As the film plays, it sounds like we are underwater. Some of these faces are asymmetrical. Some of these faces are pale and have patches of unpigmented skin while others are streaked in scars. In many of these images, people lovingly gaze at one another, embrace each other's faces, and kiss each other's cheeks. Touch here is gentle. As I rewatch this, I remember Sammie Ablaza Wills's Movement Generation's Course Correction webinar; perhaps this is what it looks like to love ourselves and one another with compassion and tenderness, like the plants.

In this montage, we are drawn in and asked to stare. We are asked to hold space. As an extension of crip erasure and ableism, as an extension of nondisabled supremacy's restrictive hold on beauty, we have been taught to look away from physically disabled bodyminds.[145] We stare at disability, at what Disability Studies scholar Rosemarie Garland-Thomson calls "extraordinary-looking bodies," because they challenge and trouble our normative expectations.[146] This film mobilizes an agentic crip beauty in the ways it invites the performers in the film to stare back at the camera and at us. Although staring as a transaction often disempowers, for Rosemarie the moment when disabled folks stare back offers a revisionary and empowered exchange.[147] Here, we as viewers are being asked to recognize crip beauty's variance: it is multidimensional, fractal, and always in becoming.

When exploring crip beauty as communal, Sins Invalid community member and activist Mordecai Cohen Ettinger writes that crip beauty is "intrinsically relational—[it] is lived, breathed, shared, and cocreated."[148] Rather than erase the innate beauties of our disabled bodyminds, crip beauty is a mutual, cooperative, cocreation of crip visibility. Sins Invalid's art-activism guides us toward witnessing all disabled, queer of color bodyminds as valid and radiant. They ask us to engage in crip beauty's reclamation of the stare so that we can render our bodyminds evidence and rewrite the majoritarian stories that have been told about us. Performing crip beauty in this way moves us past crip erasure and toward bodymind liberation.

We evolve when we create and embrace authentic representations of our disabled, queer of colour bodyminds. To find evidence of our potential for change-making, for signifying more than what the medical model of disability dictates, ensures that we can and that we are crafting our own bodymind identities and futures. In finding evidence, we embolden ourselves to enact the strategies that storytelling and recognition offer us.

CHAPTER 6

Education
Bringing Us Home

Education is how we, as disabled queer of color bodyminds, move ourselves toward collective, communal awakenings. It is how we, in defiance, learn to reclaim our bodymind autonomies and histories. Education has and will always be the constant love-action moving us closer and closer toward a practice of justice and freedom.[149] This liberatory framing positions education as the platform that can give our bodyminds the language to learn, understand, and challenge the dehumanization that has so forcefully been placed on our disabled, chronically ill, queer, trans, gender nonconforming bodyminds of color.[150] Education can help us find ourselves outside of oppressive frameworks, and it can guide us toward the creation and maintenance of crip-centric liberated zones.

Brazilian educator Paulo Freire frames education as a tool for liberation in *Pedagogy of the Oppressed*. He defines his revolutionary framework as "a pedagogy which must be forged with, not for, the oppressed (whether individuals or peoples) in the incessant struggle to regain their humanity."[151] I lean on his language here, imagining spaces where education emboldens us toward change, toward—as Disability Justice advocates—movement together. Sins Invalid educates from this place of commitment and love.[152] From this place, education becomes, as Paulo urges, "a practice of freedom."[153] Education as a practice of freedom, as progress rooted in love, grows within us a desire to celebrate the knowledge-creation of those most marginalized, *by* those most marginalized. It opens space for the purpose of growth and conversation. Education rooted in love[154] is a place where we—the disabled, queer of color many—are empowered to take ownership of our bodymind stories, our histories, and our contemporary revolutionary movements, leaders, and ancestors. Love becomes an invitation tool that galvanizes us to construct crip-centric liberated zones that help us move toward our collective liberation. In a world that tries to erase our bodyminds in the most literal of ways, Sins Invalid's educational platforms provide us with places of affirmation.

Education as Defiance

I think about Sins Invalid's cultural programming and educational platforms as an educator, which is why I arrive again and again to Paulo Freire's words, to bell hooks's *Teaching Community* and *Teaching to Transgress*, and to Bettina Love's book *We Want to Do More Than Survive*. I think about how educators of color, feminist and queer educators, disabled educators, and abolitionist educators help us to challenge what teaching can do past its white supremacist, ableist, and cis-heteropatriarchal framings; they can guide us toward something that is altogether revolutionary.

In describing abolitionist education in particular, Bettina writes that education is about "mattering, surviving, resisting, thriving, healing, imagining, freedom, love and joy."[155] This line calls to me and creates the lens through which I explore Sins Invalid's educational offerings.[156] In Bettina's description, education creates the possibility for imagining futures that are at once healing and resisting; it can provide us with the tools needed to access the liberatory narratives, lives, and histories of our bodyminds. Sins Invalid extends abolitionist education's project of "freedom, love, and joy" to also consider lessons from the lives of disabled, queer, trans, and gender nonconforming bodyminds. They extend this to all the invisiblized and disempowered people in our communities who carry the language, knowledge, and direction necessary for our collective freedom.

———————

What does it look like to create cripped, queered, decolonial education that begins from our bodymind experiences and travels outward? What does it mean to access education that heals us and grounds us back in our resilience? For Sins Invalid, this defiant education begins with Disability Justice. Their 2017 *No Body is Disposable* video series created in collaboration with the Barnard Center for Research on Women, in particular, answers these questions. Patty Berne is in conversation with Stacey Milbern, now a crip ancestor. Both activists are sitting on their wheelchairs, facing each other in Patty's home.

The first recording, "Ableism is the Bane of my Motherfuckin' Existence," introduces and explains ableism from a place of embodiment. Stacey and Patty address shame as well as the interpersonal and systemic expressions of ableism. I often use this recording in class when explaining to my students what ableism *does*. For some, this is the first time they are learning about the word. It is the first time they are beginning to understand the medical industrial complex as a system of control and power that is linked to nondisabled supremacy; it is the first time they realize how aggressively the normative, nondisabled bodymind enters into every part of our society.

Stacey begins the conversation by sharing memories from child-hood, memories of being forced to walk instead of using a wheelchair, memories of going to physical therapy and having surgeries to "fix" the aesthetic appearance of her body. She asks Patty, "is medicine about quality of life or is it about social control and perpetuating this idea of like, a good body?" I am always motivated by Stacey's question and the transformative openings it creates. Grounded in Disability Justice, she prompts us toward reconsideration: what is, in fact, a "good" body? What color is a "good" body? How does a "good" body walk, talk, think, and listen?

Stacey's question also asks us to travel in another direction. Whom does a "good" body privilege and whom does a "good" body exclude? This is the purpose of education: as we move toward reclaiming our histories and our bodymind stories, as we move toward our collective liberation, we must question, trouble, and disrupt everything we have been taught about ourselves and our communities. Returning to Paulo's *Pedagogy of the Oppressed*, as we work in all our activist movements to reclaim our collective humanity, we engage in the radical act of learning *and* unlearning; we engage in the radical act of education and knowl-edge sharing.[157]

Patty illustrates this troubling when she/they respond to Stacey by reversing the ableist comment she/they hear most frequently: "I'm so sorry that you're disabled!" Patty begins this way: "Ableism is the bane of my motherfuckin' existence. Ableism is ... it's funny because people are like, 'oh, I'm so sorry that you're disabled.' And it's absurd! I kind of want people to be like, 'I'm so sorry that we live in ableism and I'm perpetuating it every day.' Like, that's an appropriate thing to feel shitty about!" Patty pivots away from a rhetoric of shame and pity by focusing on what Paulo names as "problem-posing education."[158] For him, this type of learning and shifting asks us to question what we know and what we have been taught: "In problem-posing education, people develop their power to perceive critically *the way they exist* in the world *with which* and *in which* they find themselves; they come to see the world not as a static reality, but as a reality in process, in transformation."[159] How would our perceptions of disability change if we did not use an ableist framework? How would our perceptions of disability change if we viewed it through a Disability Justice lens? What futures, what trans formations, could we cultivate?

Problem-posing education centers asking and, in that asking, empowers us to interpret our realities as fluid places that thrive on potential. This place encourages us, as Stacey and Patty demonstrate, to depart from nondisabled supremacy and from normative knowledge systems that silence and invisibilize our bodyminds. Education and unlearning can center us again as our brazen and bold selves.

Education as Awakening

Education also serves as an awakening, as a pathway to new frameworks. In Sins Invalid's second video, "My Body Doesn't Oppress Me, Society Does," Patty and Stacey address the medical and social models of disability and the ways in which society oppresses disabled bodyminds. Patty begins by stressing that our oppressions do not come from simply being disabled: "What oppresses us is living in a system which disregards us, is violent towards us, essentially wants to subjugate our bodies or kill us. That's oppressive. My body doesn't oppress me, my body … my body's fun! But society, that can be incredibly oppressive."

I highlight this portion of the video because so much is happening here. On the one hand, Patty provides us with a critical shift: our environments—not our bodyminds—disable us. On the other hand, Patty acknowledges that it is once we are aware of this systemic oppression that we are then able to realize our disabled bodymind joys: "My body doesn't oppress me, my body … my body's fun!" This crip knowledge arouses and excites. It provokes us away from the ableist narratives that our disabled bodyminds are defective and desexual and it instead awakens us toward a liberatory framework of bodymind joy, playfulness, and autonomy. Patty and Stacey's awakening asks us to consider what would happen if we, like Aurora Levins Morales argues, realize that there is "no neutral body from which our bodies deviate." What futures could we imagine from this reframing? What new connections of self and communal love could we manifest?

Education as awakening affords us with the ability to make and remake our realities.[160] At the end of this second recording, Patty communicates the changes that need to take place: "There are always going to be crips. There are always going to be people in pain. It's just the nature of being a body. The social body we can change, and I think it requires a power analysis." This is one of the main goals of Sins Invalid's educational practice: to use a power analysis to change the normative social body, its beliefs, and its regulations. In our crip-centric liberated zones, the most marginalized among us can analyze, detangle, and speak back to the power structures that no longer serve us. This skill comes from Disability Justice's political strategies and disabled, queer of color analyses that frame all our bodyminds as valuable and as deserving of a radical, liberatory life.

In their third and final recording in collaboration with Barnard, Sins Invalid produced "The Ability to Live: What Trump's Health Cuts Mean for People with Disabilities." Here, Patty and Stacey talk about the impacts that Donald Trump's cuts to Medicaid will have on the disability community. This conversation is key for everyone to hear, particularly nondisabled folks. There is so much fear, aggravation, and uncertainty wrapped up in who deserves to access healthcare and community-setting services, what Patty calls the "basic rights to life." It is a new realization for some that disabled communities, particularly disabled bodyminds who are queer, gender nonconforming, trans and of color, are still forced to contend with the reality that they are viewed and treated—to use Patty's language—as not "viable" or worthy of life. It is a new realization for some that the eugenics principles from the twentieth century persist. Embodied/enminded knowledge shared from this place activates and incites protest. This video particularly teaches us how the lived experiences, activisms, and knowledges of our most marginalized and impacted communities can animate us toward changing the political and social body. Oftentimes, awareness is the first step in this process.

Sins Invalid's political education collaboration with the Barnard Center for Research on Women serves as an entry point. The recordings are accessible for free on Sins Invalid's website, and they are also listed on Barnard's YouTube channel. Self-described as a center that is "committed to critical feminist engagement with the academy and world," the Barnard Center's partnership with Sins Invalid introduces their intersectional community of feminist and transnational feminist scholars to Disability Justice and, by extension, Sins Invalid's body of art-activist work. This is what political education achieves for the performance project: it circulates within and beyond the community, increasing knowledge about ableism, Disability Justice, and the intersectional systems of oppression that regulate the lives and bodyminds of disabled, queer of color community. Political education teaches us to defy and challenge norms; it is an expansion of education that provokes change-making from an inherently crip, queer of color location.

Creative Workshops and Trainings

Just as Sins Invalid's political education work concentrates on the collective liberation and recognition of a phenomenally cripped future where thought and education are repositioned outside of ableism and nondisabled supremacy, their creative workshops and trainings extend this work. Their workshops emphasize the spaces we can create when we transgress ableist, racist, cis-heteropatriarchal norms. To define transgression, in the spirit of education, I turn back to bell hooks: "Urging all of us to open our minds and hearts so that we can know beyond the boundaries of what is acceptable, so that we can think and rethink, so that we can create new visions, I celebrate teaching that enables transgressions—a movement against and beyond boundaries. It is that movement which makes education the practice of freedom."[161] Transgression here is productive. It is an embodied opening inviting us to "think and rethink" so that we can make our way forward, together. This is Sins Invalid's goal as a performance project: to empower us to transgress and move past the boundaries and oppressive frameworks that restrict our bodyminds, to welcome us into crip-centric liberated zones where no bodymind is left behind.

The performance project practices these principles of transgression and education in their creative workshops. Whether they focus on voice work, poetry, movement, or crip flirting, these workshops are integral parts of Sins Invalid's cultural programming and movement building work. Grounded in Disability Justice, these events are accessible and are often offered for free to the community. These workshops have become spaces that move us out of isolation and toward a new framing of disabled bodymind expression and experience that transgresses ableism's limitations of us. However momentary and transitory, these creative workshops guide attendees toward experiencing crip-centric teaching, living, and bodymind honoring.

The Sins Invalid artist-activists that facilitate these workshops practice Disability Justice as action and as sustainable love practice. The movement-based workshops, in particular, create an expressive language demonstrating what the disabled bodymind can do. Artist Rodney Bell, for example, has offered the dance workshop "Moving in Grace" and Laura Malpass and Patty created and taught the movement workshop "Reaching for Each Other: Movement Offerings across Abilities." These facilitators crip movement and dance, transgressing the ableist assumptions that disabled bodyminds *cannot*: we cannot dance, we cannot speak through movement, we cannot express beauty in our bodyminds. Instead, participants learn that these limitations on movement and dance are not necessarily coming from *their* bodyminds, but rather from ableism's finite imagination of who can dance and of whose movement is deemed beautiful.

Sins Invalid's writing and storytelling workshops similarly advocate for transgressions, but they also emphasize self-discovery. Led by artists and Sins Invalid performers like Leroy F. Moore Jr., Maria Palacios, Nomy Lamm, and Lezlie Frye, the poetry, songwriting, and storytelling workshops encourage participants to consider the political and transformative potentials of their bodymind stories. I return to Sins Invalid's commitment to storytelling here, to their reliance on bodymind storytelling as activism, as memory, and as crip love. All these creative workshops move disabled, queer of color community to resist the narrative that only certain bodyminds have the privilege to create and transform the social and political body.

——————

Since their inception, Sins Invalid has connected with social justice organizations and educational institutions for their trainings and as a part of their Disability Justice capacity building work. Two thousand and nine was the first year the performance project participated in university conferences and engaged with community organizations. They facilitated three trainings on disabilities, ableism, and Disability Justice with the National Gay and Lesbian Task Force (NGLTF) in 2009. That same year, they conducted similar trainings focused on intersectionality, Disability Justice, and organizing at the Queer People of Color Conference at UC Davis, the Bioneers Conference, and UC Berkeley's Gender and Women's Studies Colloquia Series.

Beginning in 2010, Sins Invalid continued their Disability Justice trainings by developing their partnership with the Disability Justice Collective.[162] They extended their cross-movement solidarity work and outreach by organizing Disability Justice trainings throughout the

San Francisco Bay Area and beyond. Since their inception, Sins Invalid has worked with intersectional communities, including the Rainbow Grocery Cooperative, Phat Beets, Critical Resistance, the Brown Boi Project, the Audre Lorde Project, Queers for Economic Justice, Southerners on New Ground, Catalyst Project, and the First Nations Collective.

Most recently, in 2017 Sins Invalid began developing a relationship with San Francisco Women Against Rape (SFWAR). Aware of the incredibly high rates of physical and sexual violence against the disability community, they began working with SFWAR to ensure that they could adequately support disabled sexual assault survivors. Guided by the work of Alice Wong and Dolores Tejada, the collaboration with SFWAR began with hashtag DisabledResilient, a Twitter chat for disabled survivors of sexual assault. During the Twitter conversation, many respondents shared that they wished disability organizations had support available for survivors of sexual assault and, conversely, that organizations that support survivors focused on the specific needs of the disability community.

To establish and vocalize needs, particularly from an intersectional place, demonstrates the change-making that can happen when education's goal is to defy, resist, and awaken. After this initial Twitter conversation, Sins Invalid and SFWAR continued their cross-movement building work and developed an outreach campaign in 2018 in the Bay Area. As documented on their timeline in *Skin, Tooth, and Bone*, Sins Invalid worked with SFWAR to raise awareness of disabled survivors of sexual violence with posters throughout Bay Area transit hubs. This collaboration sought to bring visibility to survivors who are often unacknowledged and ignored.

Sins Invalid explicitly includes education as a key part of their performance project. Led by the most marginalized, these workshops, panel presentations, and collaborations intensify disabled, queer of color knowledge-making. As educational events that are also offered to a larger nondisabled community, Sins Invalid's work motivates us to transgress what we have been taught about disabilities. In understanding what this kind of awakening can do, I return to bell hooks and her definition of transgression. She writes that transgressive education "urg[es] all of us to open our minds and hearts so that we can know beyond the boundaries of what is acceptable, so that we can think and rethink, so that we can create new visions."[163] In moving us beyond, as bell hooks writes, Sins Invalid's Disability Justice–led education empowers us to build education beyond the ableist, racist, cis-heteropatriarchal narratives we have so often been given. With this type of education, we can work together to create a most loving and willfully defiant world where all our bodyminds thrive together in movement.

CHAPTER 7

Crip Kinship and Cyber Love

Many of us live, create, and connect with our crip kin from our homes. Leah Lakshmi Piepzna-Samarasinha (she/they) begins *Care Work* by naming this place of cozy crip existence and knowledge creation: "When I moved to Oakland in 2007, I started writing from bed. I wrote in old sleep pants, lying on a heating pad, during the hours I spent in my big sick-and-disabled femme of color bed cave."[164] Many of us in our crip homes create bed caves, sacred soft places where we sleep, eat, and work. We enshrine ourselves in these tender places. Sometimes we rest, exhausted, while at other times our crip homes are where we create and engage with our communities.

This ritual nesting is a part of what Leah calls our "crip emotional intelligence," the strategies and skills that we have come to know as integral to our survival. One important piece of crip emotional intelligence is her/their acknowledgement that "beds are worlds. Houses are worlds. Cars are worlds."[165] For so many of us, our beds, cars, and homes are not temporary, transitional places we inhabit for a few hours. Instead, they are the places that tether us; they are our connection to our communities. Our computers and our phones become the crip-centric liberated zones that ensure that we continue to exist in community with one another when we are too tired, too sick, and too depressed to leave.

Some of us in need of this bridging are disabled and chronically ill; others are navigating the finite resources of time and money. Regardless of where we come from and what our world looks like, we all deserve connection and access to crip-centric liberated zones. We all need an electronic entryway into a place where we can exist resilient, as our full selves. In response to this lived reality, this desire and seeking, Sins Invalid makes much of their cultural programming available online. Here, home becomes an expansive place, hundreds of thousands of miles wide. Home becomes Sins Central, becomes global viewing parties where we all teleport to performances in San Francisco. Home becomes the dance floor for a cripped out dance party, becomes space for learning. This type of digital home and community space, for so many of us, becomes our sanctuary.

Finding Crip Kinship Online

Crip-centric liberated zones that occupy cyberspace create something that we, isolated and lonely in our rooms, on our beds, on our sofas, or in our cars, need: crip kinship. Crip kinship is a network of reciprocity, a relationality that brings us closer to one another. Beyond the biological nuclear family network, kinships are informed by Indigenous and queer community knowledge.[166] They are intersectional systems, tendrils extending and creating junctions and openings for us to enter.[167] Kinship systems can help us exist in solidarity and in community. In her essay "Crip Kin, Manifesting," Alison Kafer explores crip kin as "a site of power, friction, and potentiality."[168] What calls to me most about this piece is Alison's insistence that this kinship system can be a force of change-making, that it can unsettle and challenge the ableist narratives that get told about our disabled bodyminds.

Crip kin can also forge connections between us and memory, between us and the legacy of crip resilience. Lilac Vylette Maldonado (she/they) is a sick, disabled, neurodivergent, two-spirit, Chicanx femme. As a Disability Justice activist and the cofounder and logistics coordinator of the Los Angeles Spoonie Collective, I asked her/them to speak about the importance of engaging with crip kin online:

> Online spaces, blog posts, and zines replace brick and mortar spaces never available to us. They struggle to hold our expansive collective grief while simultaneously brimming with our collective joy and healing. Here at our rich intersections of identity, in the privacy of our DMs perhaps, or in frantic posts reaching out for support, we cultivate our families where belonging and comfort are offered in exchange for solidarity. Over the frayed threads of the web, a framework for survival has been lovingly yet imperfectly created by those of us who are brave enough to imagine a kinder, better, freer world than the one we inherited. This is the framework of our kinship, it is our breadcrumb trail to liberation.

For Lilac, digital crip kin resists ableist, racist, cis-heteropatriarchal frameworks that isolate our disabled, queer of color bodyminds; in particular, digital crip kin reinserts us in community in ways that tangible spaces cannot. Its combination of intimacy and privacy gift us with, as Lilac writes, "a framework for survival that has been lovingly yet imperfectly created by those who are brave enough to imagine a kinder, better, freer world than the one we inherited." Perhaps this is the importance of cripped digital spaces: within them we are given the opportunity to move toward solidarity, however imperfect, messy, and glorious it is.

Digital space also asks us to consider what it would be like to be in relation with fellow crip kin. How could we push against and revise ableism's insistence that we are damaged? What intimacies could we alternatively craft with one another? I write the word intimacies here thinking past the word as something sexual. I think of intimacy in the way that decolonial and Indigenous scholar Dr. Kim TallBear describes during an interview for the podcast *For the Wild* in February 2020. Informed by the knowledge of asexual polyamorists in her community, Kim shares that intimacy can be "being in good relation … [intimacy] is conversation … is sharing resources, is talking to one another, listening to one another, reassuring one another. Sex can be one among many ways of relating." When I envision what crip kinship can look like and what spaces it can create, I think about Kim's definitions of intimacy and how we, in our crip kinship systems, can be in good relation with one another. Good relation is asking what someone's access needs are, what someone's pronouns are. Good relation is pod mapping, spoon check-ins, and care work. Good relation is understanding the collective access that is needed for all of us to thrive.

Making Connections: Conversations Within and Between Communities— Sins Invalid's annual, by-invitation-only community outreach series—is a journey toward achieving crip kinship, toward developing a crip intimacy sustained by conversation and resource sharing, by acknowl- edging and remembering. Our bodyminds need; our bodyminds have longing. Disability Justice's call for cross-movement and cross-disability solidarity, Disability Justice's call for collective liberation, are all possible because crip kinship and the networks it creates exist. This is endurance magic. This is survival magic, what Patty was calling on when she/they reflected on Jerika Bolen's life story. How, for example, might Jerika's understanding of her bodymind, her experience, and her life journey have shifted if she had been surrounded by crip kin, either in real time or in cyberspace? Crip kinship creates intimate networks that remind us that our bodyminds are worthy of living, that we are in community with other resilient crips chronically ill, disabled, and Mad as we are.

––––––––––

As an extension of their movement building work and as a development of crip kinship, *Making Connections* began in 2011. This online space brings community together to listen, trust, and talk through intersectional topics that most impact disabled, queer of color bodyminds. As a crip-centric liberated zone, *Making Connections* transforms our homes, our beds, and our sofas into hubs of interconnectivity, survival, and resilience. Surrounded by our warmest blankets, our snacks, tinctures, and pillows, we are empowered to connect with our communities. Sins Invalid introduces the series as a bringing "together [of] political artists, and movement-building allies involved with radical social justice projects to cross-pollinate our politically and creatively informed works."[169] As a crip-centric liberated zone, *Making Connections* becomes a communal space where we can generate and politicize crip kinship.

When *Making Connections* first began in the summer of 2011, twenty-two participants joined in cross-community dialogue, in the establishing of good relations. Since its inception, the group has explored topics that have ranged from disability and the gaze, crip spirituality, capitalist constructions of disability, ableism and language, disability and leadership, to how we can mobilize to ensure the survival of all our bodyminds after the 2016 elections, and intimate partner violence. Before each gathering, participants receive an email with questions to consider as well as written and visual resources meant to support a range of familiarity and knowledge with the topic at hand. When I first attended *Making Connections* in 2016, many participants during the Zoom call were at Sins Central. Other community members, myself included, logged on from our crip dens. In true Disability Justice fashion, we introduced ourselves, our pronouns, and our access needs before responding to the guiding questions, resource sharing, developing strategies, and holding space for our thoughts and fears. From our homes, we collaborated, we brainstormed, and we developed solutions in response to the 2016 election year. Surrounded by the glow of our computers, we found ourselves moving forward and goal setting in community. We were no longer alone.

Crip Bits: Crip Kinship as Generative Mess

In order to expand the intimate conversations that *Making Connections* encourages to the public at large, Sins Invalid began *Crip Bits* in 2017, a bimonthly conversation on Facebook. I attended many of these episodes live and got to see the questions and comments that poured into the chat box. Patty hosts the themed conversations with fellow disabled, queer of color community from her/their home in Berkeley, California. Artists, activists, and organizers, some of whom are Sins Invalid performers and community members, gather with Patty to address the issues that most affect the disability community, intersectional and rebellious as it is. As I sit at my desk, I scroll through the recorded episodes on Sins Invalid's

Facebook page. Each of these episodes is approximately one hour long. Each is live captioned and archived online on Facebook, YouTube, and on the performance project's website for easy access.

One of my favorite aspects of *Crip Bits* is the realness and the messiness of each recording. Mess is hardly negative here; it is generative. Mess is the integration and the clashing of ideas.[170] In a Disability Justice context, the mess is the real lived experiences of our bodyminds, the unplanned for and unexpected things, the moments when our needs clash against ableism's polished nondisabled mandates of how we should conduct interviews. Leah describes this clearly when she/they say that "you know you're doing [Disability Justice] because people will show up late, someone will vomit, someone will have a panic attack, and nothing will happen on time because the ramp is broken on the supposedly 'accessible' building ... Disability Justice, when it's really happening, is too messy and wild to really fit into traditional movement and nonprofit industrial complex structures, because our bodies and minds are too wild to fit into those structures."[171]

I think of this reality, the messiness of our bodyminds, as the moments of inventiveness. I see this happening over and over in the spaces Sins Invalid inhabits. In *Crip Bits* it begins with pauses, with checks to see if the Communication Access Realtime Transcription (CART) is working. Sometimes, when it is not, a viewer will type in the chat box to let the presenters know that there is a glitch. Sometimes, the conversation pauses for the live captioners. The lived reality of our disabled bodyminds and the care of crip kinship takes place in front of the camera: interviewees share that they need to take breaks because of overstimulation; Patty takes a moment on camera to ask her/their attendant to close a door; presenters take breaks to honor hunger and thirst, to stim, and to make access support requests for arm and hand adjustments; off camera, attendants bring eyeglasses and glasses of water. I think about Leah's framing of messiness and wildness here. Instead of sanitizing these crip moments with edits, *Crip Bits* shows the messiness and wildness of our bodyminds. We are shown that our bodymind access needs are radical and should be shared proudly, that they should be integrated into our daily practice of living without apology. *Crip Bits* shows that sustainability and communicating sustainability are liberatory acts. We are messy. Our needs and our expressions press against nondisabled supremacy's mandate of bodymind perfection, togetherness, and productivity, and we, instead, show ourselves as the boisterous beings that we are.

Compared to *Making Connections*, *Crip Bits* creates crip kinship and community in a more expansive way. Anyone can access these recordings; anyone can ask questions live. Since it began, the bimonthly series has focused on crip aging, crip beauty, intimate partner and sexual violence, crip sex, crip kink, fat liberation, healing justice, ableism in the academy, and crip travel tips. Crip kinship here also extends and honors cross-movement solidarity. Patty speaks with activists from the healing justice, reproductive justice, and environmental justice movements, and the fat activist community. During some episodes, Patty and her/their guests interview one another. At other times, they have prewritten questions to prompt the conversation.

In these organic, messy spaces of knowledge cocreation, the goal is to develop crip-centric liberated zones, places where we can embrace consciousness raising and the decolonizing of our bodyminds toward liberation and love. During the February 2018 episode of *Crip Bits*, Patty began the conversation about kinky crip sex by talking about self-love, liberated zones, and cyberspace: "We are in ableism, we are in white supremacy … so it's not reinforced that we are the fabulous people that we are. It's something we have to work towards. It is a consciousness we have to deliver to ourselves because the culture is not delivering it to us … I need to create microcultures of love in order to experience myself as beautiful so that's what we do here, creating a liberated zone on the internet!"[172] We create microcultures of love out of necessity, out of tenderness, and out of a need for affirmation amidst the ableism, racism, and cis-heteropatriarchy that we experience. *Crip Bits* and *Making Connections* root us, the isolated many, in digital crip kinship networks that exist with the purpose of creating microcultures of love. We access these microcultures from our crip dens where we join together in communal conversations and witnessing. We join in asking: Who are the crip kin that sustain you? What messy, gloriously overgrown microcultures do you and your community create? What do you need?

Expanding the Crip Couch

There is power in beholding our disabled, queer of color selves, in being surrounded by crip kin. Disability Studies and art scholar Ann Millett-Gallant calls this "visualizing disability,"[173] the "artistic and social representation"[174] and political resonance of witnessing all of our bodyminds gathered together. Some who have the resources, funds, and the spoons for travel can go to Sins Invalid's live performances. The rest of us who, for innumerable reasons, are not able to go in person, we attend on our crip couches, in our bedrooms, or in our friends' homes. To amplify their crip-centric liberated zone, their crip love microculture, Sins Invalid began offering pay-per-view screenings of their recorded performances beginning in 2009. This initial pay-per-view screening also served as a fundraiser for the performance project, although it was in alliance with their anti-capitalist politic: the ten-dollar cost to access the screening existed on a sliding scale and no one was prevented from accessing the link due to a lack of funds.

After they launched their online screenings, 552 private viewing parties across the United States, Canada, Europe, Australia, and Taiwan logged on to watch Sins Invalid's 2009 performance. This large viewership represents the craving and desire for disabled, queer of color storytelling and performance. Since this initial fundraiser, Sins Invalid has hosted online screenings of their documentary *Sins Invalid: An Unshamed Claim to Beauty* as well as the performances *Disability Liberated* and *Birthing, Dying, Becoming Crip Wisdom*. In their 2011 promotion for the pay-per-view presentation of Sins Invalid's 2009 annual performance, people were invited to view the performance from anywhere: a living room, bathroom, basement, a favorite dive bar, a library, or lying in the backyard on the grass, anywhere that has internet access.[175] With these small gestures, we begin to realize that crip-centric liberated zones can truly be built anywhere. This is, perhaps, the goal: we can slowly begin to transform every space into a place of abundant crip-centricity.

There is radical possibility in this broadening of space and crip home, in understanding that crip-centric liberated zones can be intentionally created anywhere. There is a broadening of where and how we can surround ourselves with crip kin. To ensure that community is created intentionally, whether it is a viewing party of one or a viewing party hosted at a university, Sins Invalid emails viewing packets to participants with guiding questions and access suggestions, along with information about the performance project, the original performance poster, and the performance program; sometimes, live Q&A's with the artists and with Patty and Leroy are also available.

I think of these viewing parties as moments of awakening, as opportunities for expansion and exposure. Communities watching may be active in social justice organizing but might not be familiar with Disability Justice. Some might be witnessing disability as empowerment, beauty, and sexiness for the very first time, while others are in active search for crip kin wherever and however it is accessible. I think here of activist Grace Lee Boggs, especially of her closing remarks at the 2008 Allied Media Conference in Detroit, Michigan. In speaking about revolution, Grace said, "A revolution, however, requires that a people go beyond struggling against oppressive institutions and make an evolutionary/revolutionary leap towards becoming more self-conscious, more self-critical, more socially responsible human beings. In order to transform the world, we/they must transform our/themselves."[176] Here, the backyard, the bedroom, and the bathtub all become liberated zones where the difficult work of self-inquiry and, as Grace writes, self-transformation can occur. We ensure that we are engaging in cross-movement solidarity when we look inward and ask ourselves who we have forgotten and whose stories we must continue to tell. During these viewing parties, we have the opportunity to transform the ableist ways in which we have been taught to think about disabilities and disabled people. We have the opportunity to transform ourselves.

Particularly because of COVID-19, Sins Invalid began earnestly generating communal online microcultures of love in 2020. Love and community creation became *Va-Va-Voom!: A Crip Dance Party*. Held early at six p.m. Pacific Standard Time so that the largest majority of folks could attend, the April and May dance parties became celebratory spaces of crip kinship and movement.[77] Participants were invited to make song requests, turn on their cameras or leave them off, dance and move in the dark or with the lights on, and dance standing or sitting on chairs. These dance parties became spaces where the disabled, chronically ill, queer of color many could journey out of isolation, out of the uncertainty, and out of the exhaustion of February and March to spring into a sexy, fierce, loving bodymind expression. It was an opportunity to persist, to refuse to hide, and to be surrounded by the communal intimacy of crip kin.

Digital Crip Kinship During COVID-19

In October 2020, in the midst of the COVID-19 pandemic, Sins Invalid livestreamed a full-length annual evening of multidisciplinary performance art. Named *We Love Like Barnacles: Crip Lives in Climate Chaos*, the performance was originally scheduled to take place at the ODC Theater in San Francisco's Mission District; however, to minimize travel and to maintain social distancing, performers recorded their work in their hometowns, then these recordings were edited together. Performances were recorded at San Francisco's ODC Theater; at Copious in Ballard, Washington; at MATCH in Houston, Texas; and at Theatre Passe Muraille and Willo' Wind Farm in Toronto, Canada. This was Sins

Invalid's first complete online performance, and it came to all of us in a time of great crip need.

We Love Like Barnacles arrived when so many in our disability communities were trying to survive while experiencing overwhelming climate changes. With the wildfires in Southern and Northern California bringing apocalyptic orange skies and ash that made it difficult for us to breathe, to hurricanes and flooding, crips were feeling the impact of climate chaos. Sins Invalid realized that if they truly wanted to do Disability Justice they needed to consider the shifts that were taking place in the environment and the ways they were harming the most marginalized among us.

An hour before the event, everyone received emails welcoming them to spend time in the pre-lounge hangout: "see a photo gallery curated from past performances, listen to some crip-centered music, learn about and visit our online auction, and chat with your friends and other guests!" The email also included a link to the evening's program, as well as additional links to view the livestream with American Sign Language interpretation or with audio descriptions. Once guests logged onto the pre-lounge hangout, they were invited to explore or join the live chat.

An average of 200–250 joined for each of the evening performances—and an average of 150 joined each of the matinee screenings—to watch Sins Invalid from their crip dens. Whereas tickets for the performance project traditionally sell out during their in-person performances, this digital performance platform expanded the tangible theater, inviting a larger community to join, bear witness, and heal. With its sliding scale ticket costs—and no one being turned away for a lack of funds—Sins Invalid ensured greater financial equity. People watched on their own or in their crip pods, with kin gathering from different cities, states, and countries. They eliminated travel costs and the parking, hotel, and food costs that often come with viewing a live Sins Invalid show. This liberatory, loving act, although necessitated by a pandemic, was clearly crip.

When *We Love Like Barnacles* performer Maria Palacios was interviewed about the new format, she shared that this would be the first time she'd watch her own performance alongside the audience. In many ways, however, she said that much would remain the same: "We will bring our troops on stage. And we will leave people in awe of the fact that not only are we existing and resisting, we're surviving and creating and changing and demanding. And that's what's beautiful about it."[178]

I come back now to Lilac's offering that digital spaces of crip kinship hold our expansive, collective grief while they simultaneously brim with our collective joy and healing. In many ways, these online spaces offer us the liberation we do not have access to in real life. They create the bridges to community that we need, the intersecting roots we crave. The content of *We Love Like Barnacles* also did this work. The evening introduced us to stories of deaths, crip loss, and crip resilience in the face of Hurricane Irma in Puerto Rico and Hurricane Harvey in Texas and Louisiana. Performers spoke about having to make the choice to leave their only wheelchair behind before getting onto rescue boats, about being forced to mourn family from a distance, and about wondering what breathing and living in the future with climate chaos will look like.

At the end of the evening, during her performance "Crip Prophesies," Maria reminded all crips watching and listening that "we will always exist," that one day, the nondisabled will become disabled, and that they will rely on our collective disabled knowledges for their continued survival. I think about the expansive online network of crip kinship that Sins Invalid has built. I think, especially, of the disabled knowledge and movement building work they have gathered, saved, and archived online. In saying "we will always exist," Maria grounds us in the good relations that come from crip kinship. This is the disabled, queer of color guidance that we are seeking. This is the magic Sins Invalid and other Disability Justice communities will offer in love and welcoming to the newly disabled. We willfully persist, to return to Sara Ahmed. Despite every ableist, racist, cis-heteropatriarchal attempt at erasure, we are not going anywhere.

CHAPTER 8

Crip Sex as Transformative Pleasure Universe

To crip sex is to provoke, to break open, to unsettle. To crip sex disturbs the normative belief that nondisabled, heteronormative sex is always the default.[179] In this new universe, this burst, crip sex opens futures of possibilities where we can hold the words "sex" and "disability" on our tongues without resistance; it centers the wisdom and activism of the disabled, queer of color community who are in search of transformative change. Here, crip sex is an offering, an atlas guiding us back to the inherent knowing that our bodyminds deserve pleasure, bliss, and contentment. Crip sex helps us create liberatory frameworks that welcome our disabled, queer of color bodyminds in all their lusciousness.[180]

For over a decade, pleasure and sexuality have been a part of Sins Invalid's Disability Justice politics as well as their artmaking and educational platforms. In their crip-centric liberated zones, we learn to unmake the oppressive limits that are artificially placed around sex, desire, and pleasure. In this tender and seductive place of declaration, Sins Invalid's multimedia performances position our bodyminds as desire: bodies

embracing and washing each other on stage, stories of masturbation as
pain management and self-love, and a wheelchair striptease, all sexy and
hungering, all needed, all made commonplace. Crip sex is more than
sex, more than embodiment; crip sex stewards a reconstruction of sex.[181]

————

Within the political imaginary of crip sex, disabled, queer of color community acknowledge their sexual agency.[182] From this cripped place,
we can reframe sex as a "civil and political right"[183] and as a decolonial
and queer project that severs, challenges, deconstructs, and opens
up new ways to conceptualize sex. In this crip-centric liberated zone
informed by Disability Justice, choice and bodily autonomy fracture the
racist and colonial lineages of sterilization abuses in the US: the nonconsensual sterilizations of predominately immigrant, poor, Spanish-
speaking Latinx women at County USC Medical Center in the 1970s;
the Mississippi "appendectomies" that sterilized poor Black women and
girls in the South from the 1920s to the1960s; and "la operación" in
Puerto Rico and in the East Coast of the US that sterilized Puerto Rican
women and girls in the 1960s. Crip sex's offering of choice and bodily
autonomy resists the frameworks of compulsory heterosexuality and
heterosexism: the violence of conversion therapy and the over seven
hundred thousand LGBTQ community members who were subjected
to it;[184] the pathologizing of homosexuality in the *Diagnostic Statistical
Manual of Mental Disorders* (DSM) until 1973, and the current pathologizing of gender dysphoria. When we enter into a sexual worldview
that is at once crip, queer, and decolonial, we can imagine new ways to
restore our full humanity.

In thinking about crip sex and the crip sexual culture that Sins Invalid inhabits and fosters, I keep returning to adrienne maree brown's inventive and nourishing framework of pleasure in her book *Pleasure Activism*. Pleasure activism calls on us to view all expressions of pleasure—not just the erotic —as decolonizing acts of reclamation: the gratification of sitting in the sun, of surprising someone at work or home, of floating in water, or of stroking the roundness of our bellies. adrienne argues that our empowerment roots our exploration and manifestation of pleasure. She writes, "Pleasure activism asserts that we all need and deserve pleasure and that our social structures must reflect this. In this moment, we must prioritize the pleasure of those most impacted by oppression."[185] It is a revelation to embrace and foreground pleasure, particularly for those of us who are most often most distanced from it.

By honoring the pleasure of those most marginalized, those more distanced from pleasure, Sins Invalid moves us into an enticing, restorative place. For disabled, queer of color community, this gratifying place rewrites the shame and silencing associated with embodied pleasures, sexual autonomy, joy, and beauty. This new cripped sexual culture teaches us how to, as adrienne urges, "align our pleasures with our values."[186]

"As a person with a disability, I don't have to mimic [nondisability] in order to be sexual."

Over the last twelve years, Sins Invalid has created crip-centric liberated zones that move disability and sex past the restrictive territory of incongruence and disconnection.[187] In their cripping of pleasure, sex, and eroticism, the performance project unearths the history of sexual trauma, silence, and the polarizing narratives that impact so many in our disabled, queer of color communities. Sometimes our bodyminds are forced to navigate the stereotypes of infantilization and desexuality. At other times, we are forced into the opposite and are hypersexualized and fetishized. And still, at other times, we are viewed as abject and disgusting, our bodyminds moved further and further away from sexuality and pleasure. To imagine a crip sexual universe *despite* these histories is to express the activist, revisionary potential of cripped pleasure, the type of pleasure that adrienne names the "orgasmic yes!" The orgasmic yes is declaration, an embodied joy that initiates activism and change. I imagine the orgasmic yes as something tangible, a sensory explosion with an earthy, salty taste. The orgasmic yes mobilizes; its urgency moves us toward changing, revising, and remembering. For Sins Invalid, the orgasmic yes was the conversation that Patty Berne and Leroy F. Moore Jr. had over dinner at La Peña. It was Patty's declaration that they should create their own venue where they could collectively work toward unlearning shame and enacting a uniquely queer and of color crip sexual liberation.

In an interview with Cory Silverberg, Patty clarifies Sins Invalid's focus on sexuality by saying:

> Sins Invalid is not just about saying "We're sexual too!"—clearly, we are sexual too—but it's about how we do crip sex, how do we have sex and view it erotically through the lens of disability. It's similar to the struggle that we may experience as people of color when we endeavor to "decolonize our minds" and stop whitewashing ourselves ... As a person with a disability, I don't have to mimic [nondisability] in order to be sexual. I can experience my sexuality as crip, as someone who fully occupies a

non-normative physical space. And part of that movement to full living in one's own experience is naming and resisting dehumanization. So, all of that has to be in the show. It's life, so it's in the show.[188]

For Sins Invalid, the spaces they create liberate sex from the ableist myth that only nondisabled people can be sexual and have children. What is most powerful for me in Patty's reflection is her/their claim that they do not need to "mimic [nondisability] in order to be sexual." This is what recognition and healing gifts us: a movement toward sexuality as a human right. It is a distancing from comparison, from the mythology of a "good" body, from the mythology that there is only one way to have sex. Patty introduces us to an empowered, cripped sexual universe where sex is no longer restricted to the genitals or even to touching. Every orifice, every body part is renewed, lusting, and full of potential. Here, sex becomes glorious at times, awkward in others, an act of conversation and a pause, and always a journey of negotiation and communication. Rather than mimic nondisabled sex, crip sex resists assumptions about sex, what it looks like, or what a partner might or might not desire. Crip sex becomes pleasure, voluminous and all-embracing.

———————

When I think of what crip sexuality creates, I think of Cara Page's opening poem as the MC at Sins Invalid's 2009 performance at the Brava Theater. Cara walks onstage wearing a black skirt and corset and knee-high boots; a brown fur drapes over her shoulders. She begins the evening with an emboldened, sensual offering: "Welcome to our queendom, kingdom, queerdom, multibodied universe ... Tonight, we will be new maps of celestial beings, new constellations setting course for our collective bodies and shapes to create what freedom and love can look like, taste like, without any perfect body, any perfect shape, or form, without assuming any single way of thinking or desire. There is no right or wrong body of a conscious, revolutionary mind. Tonight, we will show you the many ways we come as alchemists of truth and change toward accepting that each of us are perfectly scarred."

Cara declares possibility. Her words serve as map, as routing. They welcome us into a place where the pleasure of crip-centricity has the potential to move us away from limitations, particularly the limitations of nondisabled desire. Her poem resculpts the Brava Theater as a crip-centric liberated zone, a "constellation setting course" for new, perhaps unexplored sexual pleasure terrains. In this place, the oppressions dictated by the "perfect body" do not exist, nor do the assumptions surrounding desire and sexuality.

As I rewatch this beginning, this invitation, I return to adrienne's call for pleasure activism, to her declaration that pleasure has the capacity to "shift[t] the ground beneath us, inside us, and transforming what is possible between us."[189] Sins Invalid's crip-centric liberated zones ask us to similarly engage in shifting our imaginations both internally and communally. What do desire, pleasure, and sex look and feel like outside of nondisabled supremacy? Cara's introduction extends this work by encouraging us to experience the liberation of sex.

————————

"It felt important to provide a mirror for what we needed to see in the world and to see each other as sexual and desirable and beautiful in a world that says we are not."

The so-called impossibility of crip sex in the nondisabled imaginary is not new. To emphasize this point, Sins Invalid begins their documentary, *Sins Invalid: An Unshamed Claim to Beauty*, with artist and poet Maria Palacios saying, "Sex and disability are two words that you don't often hear together, and if you do, it's like [gasp] those people have sex?"[190] In the ways that Sins Invalid explores the erasure of disabled, queer of color bodyminds—our stories, histories, and activisms—the performance project also dedicates itself to imagining a future where our bodyminds can have the choice to relish in a generative, juicy crip sexual culture; in dedicating themselves to creating a vocabulary of crip sex, Sins Invalid resists the gasp.

During the November 2017 episode of *Crip Bits*, "Fucking While Cripped," Stacey Milbern moderates a conversation between Patty and India Harville, an African American disabled queer performance artist, somatic bodyworker, activist, and Sins Invalid performer. Patty and India discuss the elements of and the need for crip sex, as well as Sins Invalid's focus on embodiment and sexuality. Stacey begins the conversation by stressing that, informed by ableism, "the social body neuters people with disabilities." She shares that for this reason, "It felt important [for Sins Invalid] to provide a mirror for what we needed to see in the world and to see each other as sexual and desirable and beautiful in a world that says we are not."[191] It is an act of protest for Sins Invalid's artist-activists to present their bodyminds as adventurous, sexy, and lusting. It is a liberatory act to create an alternative, crip-centric narrative of what sex means and to have this mirrored in performances and in community spaces.

During the *Crip Bits* episode, I kept finding examples of how this metaphor of mirroring does more than reflect an inclusive representation of desirability and sexuality; mirroring also offers an expansion of what sex from an activist location can do. India expressed this clearly when she shared that during crip sex, "I can bring my whole self ... and all of the things that are sometimes hard about my body can either be celebrated or loved on or lifted up inside crip sex." Crip sex challenges all of us to reframe sex as more than just active and autonomous.[192] In this new crip sexual culture, sex is no longer contingent on a bed, on the genitals, or on penetration;[193] sex is no longer contingent on performance or on rapid movement all the time, every time. Sex and desire can be anything that our bodyminds need, anything that brings us pleasure. India describes it this way: "Sometimes I can't be touched or it's painful to be touched, and so maybe our sexual encounter begins with some sort of sexy gazing from a distance or maybe I'm going to do a striptease or something because that is going to feel good for my body and is a part of my sexuality. That is added and appreciated inside of crip sex in a way that I think sometimes non-crip sex will not be as open to."[194]

This is the celebration and uplift of crip sex and crip sexual culture: it has the potential to adjust and broaden our limited definitions of non-disabled sex. As a mirroring, it awakens us to the possibility that sex and what is viewed as erotic and pleasurable is as varied as we are. For me, one of the most radical parts of crip sex is the questions it poses: how would our conceptions of sex change if we viewed it as a civil and political right? How does nondisabled sex limit all of our bodyminds—whether we are disabled or not? What possibilities does normative sex take away from us? What expansive, accessible practices in addition to or excluding sex could crip sex open for us?

Most powerfully, crip sex amplifies and offers to us voices and thought practices from the margins. The margins are often our compost. They are not disempowered or dispossessed places. They are the ripe and fertile places we create from. We gather in all our exhausted realities to come together, tell stories, dream rebellious dreams, and create change that grows outward from this place. bell hooks writes that "radical possibility" comes from the margins: "[The margin] is also the site of radical possibility, a space of resistance. It was this marginality that I was naming as a central location for the production of counter hegemonic discourse that is not just found in words but in habits of being and the way one lives ... [the margin] nourishes one's capacity to resist. It offers to one the possibility of radical perspective from which to see and create, to imagine alternatives, new worlds."[195]

When bell hooks writes about the radical potential of margins, even though she writes about colonized and oppressed people of color, I happily stretch and apply her words to disabled communities. We, too, in our resistance build imaginative new ways to live in this world; we use our lives and experiences from the margins to create nourishment and empowerment. Sins Invalid's imagining of a crip sexual future distinctly comes from this marginal place, from this place of crip dreaming and crip envisioning. From the margins outward, the performance project creates, to return to Stacey, a mirror, a kaleidoscopic reflection of a diversely sexual pleasure universe. From the margins outward, Sins Invalid's art-activism and education create alternatives outside of white and nondisabled supremacy, outside of cis-heteropatriarchy.

Dear reader, imagine what your bodymind would move toward if your sexual pleasure universe privileged autonomy and consent, if it was not regulated by normative ideas of what it means to "be sexy" or "attractive." What feelings and sensations would your bodymind linger on? What need could you finally and lovingly satisfy?

"Sexuality is magic; it is a way that we weave ourselves into the world from the inside out."

In her 2008 performance, "Wall of Fire," Nomy Lamm (they/them) begins with the breath. They stand by a table, their arm resting on a reverb machine while their right hand holds a microphone close to their mouth. As a voice teacher, creative coach, performance artist, Kohenet Hebrew Priestess, and as Sins Invalid's creative director, Nomy's art activism imagines a crip sexual culture from the margins outward. Their performance art is about space holding just as much as it is about providing connectivity.

Nomy begins to sing: "Stroke one, two, three / Breathe one, two, three / Stroke one, two, three / Breathe one, two, three."[196] Slow and meditative, they draw us in. Their voice loops into the reverb machine until Nomy lifts the slit of their red dress. This is the first time we see Nomy's prosthesis. They lean back out of it and hold the leg in front of their body, almost as if they are presenting it to us as an offering. As they begin to use their prosthesis as a drum, Nomy renders embodiment as sound and possibility. While the first stanza loops, they continue singing, overlapping voice and percussion: "Magic breathes, and magic comes / I believe in magic theorems / Take me to your inner sanctum / I'm going

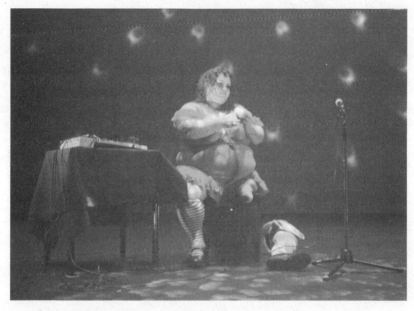

Nomy Lamm in "Wall of Fire", 2008. *Sins Invalid Annual Performance*, Brava Theater. Photo by Richard Downing, courtesy of Sins Invalid.

to watch you come / I'm going to watch you come." The music of "Wall of Fire" is sultry. This is a temptation song, a desire song. Nomy begins to delicately pull up the microphone's cord, folding it, and enticing us with a provocation of fingers. They run their hands playfully over their body, their stomach. In the face of fat phobia and the messages of sizeism our culture tries to submit us to, Nomy asserts the sensualness of the stomach, of the curve.

Nomy's performance asks that we as viewers expand and liberate our understanding of what sexuality can look like when it revels in Fat[197] cripness. When I asked Nomy about the importance of performing eroticism and sexuality as a visibly disabled person, they observed that "sexuality is magic; it is a way that we weave ourselves into the world from the inside out, and people with disabilities have to work hard to claim our sexualities so that what we are bringing into the world is powerful [and] concentrated."[198] Their dress, the removal of their prosthesis, and the repetitive loop of their voice forge a radical sexual culture for all bodyminds. Here, words like infantile, desexual, and passive lose their possessive grip. Claiming crip sexuality as magic and as incantation is one powerful way for Nomy to declare themselves present and true, particularly in an ableist, racist, cis-heteropatriarchal culture that wishes nothing more than to render their sexual embodiment invisible and invalid.

During our interview Nomy stressed the sexual agency that "Wall of Fire" harnesses, reinforcing the idea that sexuality belongs to all bodyminds: "For me being able to claim my own sexuality has meant walking into the fire in a way. There is stuff that is really scary ... to claim my own desire has been quite a process. Performance has been a ritual that I have used in my life to bring things into reality ... My leg in most of my relationships is phallic because I can fuck people with it. There is something intensely healthy about reclaiming pleasure with the parts of the body that have been medicalized."[199]

Performance is where Nomy reclaims their body, identity, and sexuality from intersecting networks of oppression. It is a place that offers them a journey into a self-crafted, self-fought-for reality where crip sexual agency is not just possible but is a necessity. Because Nomy must walk into the fire to claim their sexuality, "Wall of Fire" names the immense work that needs to take place to rewrite the desexualization that is so aggressively placed on disabled bodyminds. The third stanza of their song alludes to this: "Now I can't run and there's nowhere to hide

/ I gotta get back inside / The wall of fire is so intimidating / But I gotta get mine and I'm not waiting." In this politicized space, Nomy proclaims the Fat, crip bodymind as a desiring, radical being: the shimmy, the grace of exposed shoulders, the stroke, the arched back, and the smile.

—————

"Droolicious, baby, come here and give me kisses. Straight from my lips into your mouth. Goddam I'm making disability hot and famous."

In our cripped, pleasure universes, we have the opportunity to revisit our bodyminds and reinscribe meaning; we as sexually agentic bodyminds are emboldened with the power to rename. Sins Invalid cofounder Leroy F. Moore Jr. is an African American krip writer, poet, activist, and is the founder of Krip Hop Nation.[200] He engages in the renaming of sexuality in "Droolicious," a spoken word piece he performed at Sins Invalid's Crip Soirée in October 2013 at the Brava Theater. Leroy swagger-walks onstage and begins the performance with a moan, with a slurp, and with an exquisite roll of the tongue:

> I've got my own language
> Speaking slow fat tongue
> Scares knocking knees
> On billboards displaying body image
> Cerebral Palsy, was schooled to catch my drool
> Now I'm a man changing the rules
> Found someone who thinks it's sexy
> Now I'm naming it. Droolicious

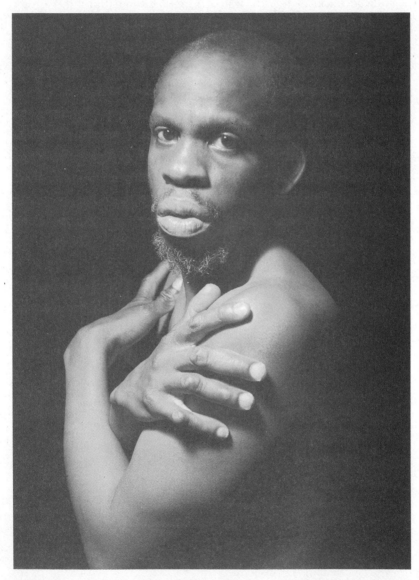

Portrait of Leroy F. Moore Jr., 2007. Photo by Richard Downing, courtesy of Sins Invalid.

Baby, come here & give me kisses
Straight from my lips into your mouth
Goddam I'm making disability hot & famous …
What a relief it is
My drool is now Droolicious
Close your eyes imagine this
Rolling down my chin onto your body
Drip drip drop drop fizz fizz.

Leroy's spoken word grounds us in a krip sexual universe that questions and rule-changes what drool means. He speaks from the margins, from a krip sexual universe of pleasure. As he speaks in his own language with his slow fat tongue, Leroy liberates drool. Rather than a source of embarrassment or shame, drool becomes the audiovisual reminder of the juiciness of krip sex. It becomes rhythmic sound and presence, something he slurp-sucks, something that leaps off stage. Here, drool becomes punctuation and diction.

In Leroy's kripped sexual universe, drool is slick and sensual invitation. During the performance, when he pauses to stress the words "baby," "goddamn," and "drool," the audience erupts with cheers and whistles. His spoken word performance actively seduces us, and the engagement is reciprocal. When Leroy says, "drip drip drop drop," drool, the lubricated erotic, forms around the sides of his lips in real time. Leroy invites the audience to wrestle with, question, and reconcile our own connotations of drool, and in doing so, we are invited to collectively cocreate an erotic where all our bodyminds are desiring and deliciously empowered. The atmosphere on the stage becomes an expression of adrienne maree brown's orgasmic yes! It is the reciprocity that only consensual, kripped sex can bring.

When I spoke to Leroy about "Droolicious" and how the performance resisted the embodied censorship of nondisabled supremacy, he shared that calling attention to drool is a sensual act of self-acceptance and recognition: "'Droolicious' is really about taking back the term drool. I looked [drool] up in the dictionary and all the definitions were [negative] so I wanted to really put my spin on it and make it sexy. It *is* sexy. I wanted to flip the notion that mainstream society has about people with disabilities." In this place of celebration, Leroy moves drool away from the lessons of self-control he was taught as a young person. Krip sexual culture here becomes a playful, uninhibited, unregulated space where we are motivated to create our own rules of embodiment.

At the end of the performance, Leroy slurp-sucks his drool before he says "droolicious" three more times. With this incantation, he forges his krip sexuality in language and sound. This unshamed krip sexual universe creates and invites us to participate; it is at once revolutionary and resistant. In all of its unruly grace, no longer medicalized and no longer desexed, drool becomes liberation and broadens the possibilities of krip pleasure.

"Liberation in the context of [Disability Justice] includes the right to sexual pleasure and choice and desire for all types of disabled people."

In both editions of *Skin, Tooth, and Bone*, the Sins Invalid community includes a chapter on sexuality. This decision extends the performance project's focus on sexual freedom by addressing the alignments between Disability Justice and sexual politics. As a political framework that advocates for progress and forward movement with no bodymind left behind, Disability Justice most certainly recognizes embodied/ enminded and interactive experiences of pleasure as necessary for liberation. I return here to adrienne's work around pleasure activism, specifically to her question, "Is it possible for justice and pleasure to feel the same way in our collective body?" To this question Sins Invalid provides a resounding and, to use adrienne's language, an orgasmic yes! In the long tradition of disabled sex educators and activists[201] and scholars, the performance project presents examples of how crip sexual desire, communication, and pleasure are in fact social justice issues.

The chapter entitled "Disability Justice and Sexuality" documents an interview conducted by journalist Cory Silverberg between Patty and NEVE Mazique (they/he), a disabled, multigendered, mixed race, Black performance artist. In its centering of disabled, queer of color lives, Disability Justice invests in acknowledging and reversing the oppressive narratives around sexuality. Patty addresses ableism's cycle of sexual oppressions by beginning the conversation with erasure: "One of the ways that disabled people are oppressed is through the negation of our sexualities as a means of denying the viability of our bodies. We can see this ... through the general public dread of what it means to expose the nude disabled body."[202] Disability Justice's goal of collective liberation reminds us that we are resilient and that all our bodyminds are worthy of celebration. We are all deserving. We all have the right to be crip pleasure-seekers. In our rebellious and expansive crip sexual cultures, we have the freedom to relish in the textures of our own bodies or in the bodies of our lovers. We can relish in the sensation of a tomato bursting in our mouths, in new growths in our gardens, or in the swift, leathery tips of a whip. Our carnal paths and our carnal loves are ours to decide.

To view crip sexuality from this place is to similarly praise the wisdom of all our bodyminds and to resist the mechanisms and legacies of sexual oppression.

———————

For NEVE, Disability Justice transforms sex far beyond ensuring accessibility. With its focus on choice, their/his framing of sex intersects with reproductive justice politics, a movement building framework that privileges a person's ability to choose their own reproductive future. Reproductive justice moves past the mainstream white feminist movement's focus on abortion rights and develops strategies for addressing the systemic inequalities that impact all reproducing bodyminds, including women, girls, gender nonconforming, and trans folks who are of color, who are immigrants, and who are disabled.[203] NEVE's discussion here pulls on themes present in both movement building frameworks. In particular, they/he stresses that ableism eradicates choice and bodily autonomy: "[Ableism is] negating our agency, our ability to make choices, and our right to make choices! An important intersection between [Disability Justice] and sexuality is the issue of choice. I think about reproductive justice and eugenics, and wonder about people's question of whether people with developmental disabilities can consent to sex. Having a [Disability Justice] lens about sexuality and consent is incredibly important because it centers the full humanity of the disabled person."[204]

Choice is powerful here. Choice and humanity interweave and become stars in our crip sexual universe; they become guideposts in our crip-centric liberated zones. Disability Justice resists assumptions around sex and desire by advocating for choice and the political spaces it actualizes.[205] Choice empowers all our bodyminds to decide for ourselves the pathways of longing and sex we wish, or do not wish, to travel upon.

––––––––––

Disabled, queer of color bodyminds: we dream sex past the margins. Normative sex expectations do not suit us, do not hold space and potential for all our cravings or for all the ways we live in wholeness and interdependence with our bodies and with our loves. So, we create something else, something more authentic and self-directed. We, in all our resilience, actualize a crip sexual culture that politicizes our bodymind needs and desires. We, together, manifest transformative crip abundances.

CHAPTER 9

Beauty as Liberation, as Splendid Crip Future

As we imagine and create crip-centric liberated zones, what will our beauty futures look like? In this decolonial place, who will we center and what norms will we finally collectively acknowledge as damaging and violent? In 2018, a roundtable conversation took place among Disability Justice and Trans Liberation activists Patty Berne, Jamal T. Lewis, Stacey Milbern, Malcolm Shanks, Alok Vaid-Menon, and Alice Wong. The community gathered to discuss Sins Invalid's crip-centric expansions of beauty. During the roundtable, Alok unpacked the nuances of the performance project's beauty practice by first discussing the oppressions of normative beauty: "Liberation is about being liberated from 'beauty' and, in turn, approaching beauty with our own terms. Beauty can be a violent system: one which sanctions whose lives matter and whose do not, one which justifies, and indeed glorifies, brutality in the name of a greater good. I but believe it is possible to reclaim beauty for ourselves, by which I mean finding ways of relating to each other outside of what we've been taught to desire."[206]

Alok's reclamation of beauty here serves as invitation, as a revolutionary, inclusive, and loving opening. If we can approach beauty on our own terms, if we can imagine beauty as liberatory and voluminous, then perhaps we can disentangle normative beauty from its violent ableist, white supremacist, and cis-heteropatriarchal restrictions.

This is, in fact, what Sins Invalid does. The performance project engages with beauty as reclamation, as agentic. Patty communicates this best when she/they say during an interview that "One of the catchphrases we [in Sins Invalid] have is that beauty always, always recognizes itself. It does. If you think that the divine is the same thing as beauty is the same thing as love, it does, it strives for itself."[207] In this framing, beauty becomes a resilient and community-driven politic. Beauty becomes self-love, becomes intervention, becomes the intense joy of finding ourselves once again without the oppressive lenses we were raised with. Beauty becomes the reminder that our bodyminds are remarkable in all their presentations and expressions.

"If age and disability teach us anything, it is that investing in beauty will never set us free."

Embedded in the conversation of Disability Justice and beauty is Mia Mingus's work on the Ugly. During the Femmes of Color Symposium in Oakland, California, in 2011, she gave a keynote address entitled, "Moving Toward the Ugly: A Politic Beyond Desirability." For Mia, the Ugly teaches us to interrogate and challenge the restrictions of normative beauty and desirability. The Ugly helps us to understand beauty as an oppressive framework informed by ableism, capitalism, consumerism, transphobia, and white supremacy. In crafting the Ugly, Mia asks that we leave beauty behind: "There is only the illusion of solace in beauty. If age and disability teach us anything, it is that investing in beauty will never set us free. Beauty has always been hurled as a weapon. It has always taken the form of an exclusive club ... I don't think we can reclaim beauty."[208] For Mia, beauty is restriction and artifice and has everything to do with ableism and the systems of oppression that regulate us. Beauty has everything to do with mandates, with restrictive binaries, with rules, and with consumerism. Beauty excludes, restrains, and causes harm. On the other hand, the Ugly, to use Mia's words, is magnificent. The Ugly asks that we engage in the difficult process of no longer apologizing for our bodyminds, that we refuse to stigmatize all the parts of us that normative society has labeled as ugly or invaluable. She reminds us that although it is difficult, we need to "Respec[t] Ugly for how it has shaped us and been exiled. Seeing its power and magic, seeing the reasons it has been feared. Seeing it for what it is: some of our greatest strength."[209]

I understand and feel so much of this keynote. I read Mia's argument that we must question and resist normative beauty culture and all of its ableist, racist, cis-heteropatriarchal damage and thought, yes! We need to have a conversation about the magnificence of Ugly, the magnificence of bodyminds that have been called "unhuman" and "undesirable" for so long.[210] I also agree that we need to reposition the caustic sting that is hurled with the use of the word ugly: ugly as an insult is projected at the bodies of our gender nonconforming loves, at the bodies of our loves of color, and at the bodies of our physically disabled loves. It degrades our community's worth and distances us from our courage, our tenacity, and our self-affirming magic. Mia argues that in order to get to a new place where we are not the casualties of a weaponized beauty culture, we need to challenge desirability politics and embrace the Ugly; we cannot, as she writes, reclaim beauty. Sins Invalid offers us a similar practice of deconstructing and distancing ourselves from normative beauty standards; however, they use a distinctly different tactic.

Sins Invalid weaves beauty, desire, and eroticism directly into their mission statement. They write that their art-activism challenges the "paradigms of 'normal' and 'sexy' ... offering instead a vision of beauty and sexuality inclusive of all bodies and communities."[211] They embrace beauty and its political potential unabashedly, so much so that their subtitle is "an unshamed claim to beauty." Sins Invalid offers us a restoration of beauty as liberation. In their multidisciplinary artmaking, they ask us to imagine a reality where we can actively detach beauty from ableism, racism, and cis-heteropatriarchy. What would it look like to enter into a space where beauty is for everyone? What would it look like, what would it feel like, to emancipate beauty? To decolonize beauty? To crip and queer beauty? What would the possibility of an intersectional, sustainable, and vulnerable beauty offer us?

Sins Invalid's goal here is similar to Mia's politicization of the Ugly. Both urge us to collectively challenge and reframe normative beauty. Both ask us to move away from a simplistic adoption of beauty and its oppressions. The difference is that Mia upholds the Ugly and the eradication of beauty as the path we should take, while Sins Invalid asks that we embark on a project of beauty restoration and salvaging. According to their framework, we arrive to a new place where, perhaps, beauty never belonged to ableism, never belonged to the restrictions of white supremacy or cis-heteropatriarchy. Sins Invalid asks us to consider beauty instead as something that existed *before*. Similar to sexuality, the performance project suggests that to create crip-centric liberated zones and collective liberation, we also must restore beauty.

"I was searching for beauty and I named myself."

Part of the politicization of disability, for Sins Invalid, is the activation of beauty as defiance and verb. During the 2018 panel discussion, "Beauty Always Recognizes Itself," Alice acknowledges that for many, the recharacterization of beauty beyond the superficial is new.[212] For Sins Invalid, creating a platform where community can witness the aesthetic, embodied, and experiential beauties of disabled, queer, gender nonconforming, and trans bodyminds of color directly resists the labels of disposability and undesirability that have been placed on these communities. She shares that this act of recognition is what fuels revolution and liberation; it is what mobilizes us to recreate ourselves in collectivity and love.[213]

For many of us, our birth is our first moment of resistance. Our birth is not necessarily the moment at which we entered this world, though it certainly can be. For many of us, we are born when we enter into the practice of self-love and affirmation; we are born as proud disabled bodyminds in the moment we find our communities, in the moment we discover Disability Justice, in the moment we understand that we are no longer alone. Here, we reconstruct beauty as activism; beauty becomes the threshold, the incandescent moment when we birth ourselves.

Sins Invalid affirms this birthing of bodymind beauty in their 2016 performance *Birthing, Dying, Becoming Crip Wisdom*. At the beginning of the evening, NEVE dances on stage from their/his wheelchair with Antoine Hunter; Hunter is a Deaf, African American, Indigenous, disabled, two-spirit dancer and choreographer. During the performance, "Bringing It Black,"[214] we hear NEVE's voice overhead as their/his arms entangle with Antoine's, as their/his arms reach and stretch and push: "My whole life it was so much easier to imagine a white, able-bodied, normatively gendered person dancing, having sex, stroking whatever it is I stroke, gesturing about whatever it is I gesture about, easier because really looking into mirrors was such a task. To be born like us, like you, like me is to be born into a world that doesn't want to offer us a reflection of ourselves or any qualifiers that will allow us to exist. How is it that you existed anyway? … I was searching for beauty and I named myself."

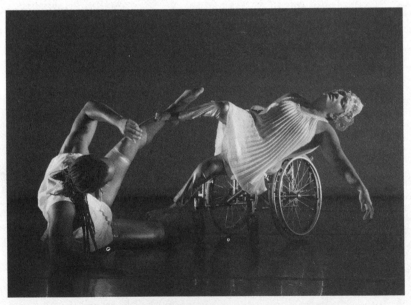

NEVE and Antoine Hunter in "Bringing It Black", 2016. *Birthing, Dying, Becoming Crip Wisdom*, ODC Theater. Photo by Richard Downing, courtesy of Sins Invalid.

We must birth ourselves, our disabled, queer of color selves, the moment we realize that we live in a world that does not value our disabilities, our gender nonconformity or queerness, when we realize that we live in a world that does not value our bodyminds. When NEVE asks how it is that we exist anyway, they/he is asking us to look inward, to search for the beauty and strength that grew us in a world that is not made for us. They/he is asking us to name ourselves in a beauty that we have always known to exist.

Part of this recognition journey, this intention to exist anyway, is the capacity, or perhaps the necessity, to birth ourselves. In birthing, NEVE asks us to consider how we affirm our bodyminds past the stereotypes and failures that are expected of us. In response to NEVE, activist and political educator Malcolm Shanks speaks while Antoine and NEVE continue to dance: "Giving birth to myself means choosing to become what I wish to be and to see myself as opposed to the frozen tropes, stereotypes, and expectations the world has pushed onto me. Coming into my gender nonconformity feels like giving birth to myself, like coming back from the fossilized. Choosing to grow out my hair, pierce my skin, paint my face feels like another example of using my body to create an anti-colonial nonhuman possibility, just like my mother's decision to give birth to me."

I think of the phrase "coming back from the fossilized" when I think of what recognition and affirmation can do, when I think of what beauty as disabled, queer of color action feels like. To say that we are bodyminds of significance and relevance is to say that we are intrinsically beautiful. It is to say that our bodymind liberation comes from resistance and from the intentional birthing of ourselves. We, as disabled, queer of color bodyminds, are emboldened with the power to transform ourselves from the fossilized expectations that are placed upon us. We can renounce; we can refuse, and that is distinctly beautiful.

During their next performance, "Welcome Back to Life," there is a brief pause as NEVE looks out onto the audience. In their/his white flowing dress and fairy crown, they/he speaks to our diverse, active beauties, what they/he calls the glowing and claiming of our lives: "It is a claim to our lives, our desires, our ecstatic being. And yes, our traumas, our cracks, our quakes, and yes, our raining shining love and yes what we leave behind that we hope others will scoop up with whatever parts scoop to rebuild the world again. To glow is not to say, to not also sag, to rest, to roll over, to reach up, to ask, to answer, to sing."

NEVE's performance splits open the normative use of the word "beauty." To claim ourselves in our beauty and rebirthing is, as they/he says, to "rebuild the world." It is the holding of our bodyminds in all their needs. NEVE expands on this rebuilding when, later in the performance, they/he rolls out onstage and names our disabled bodyminds as beautiful and revolutionary destinations: " … with your contracted elbows, vibrational hinged tongues, lips dripping music, stomachs balling fists, with your fire skin, and your twirling balletic minds." This is crip, neurodiverse, Mad beauty. It is bodymind celebration and it *is* political. Sins Invalid's performance space becomes a map of liberated beauty, an invitation that we can cocreate and arrive to a restored beauty that can help us embolden a most splendid crip future.

"I think we must decolonize ourselves, play large, know our fabulousness, our worth, our power in the face of being told that our beauty could not be."

When I think of Sins Invalid's beauty politic, I think past the physical manifestations of the aesthetic, and I think of the beauty and love that serves as the groundwork of our communities. I think again back to bell hooks and her insistence that our communities can disrupt and recreate oppressive definitions of beauty.[215] I imagine a beauty manifestation, an atlas of beauty, that is community created with all the love our disabled, queer of color universe has to give. To disrupt normative beauty is to create a magical place of bodymind reconciliation. When bell hooks writes, "Choosing love we also choose to live in community, and that means that we do not have to change by ourselves,"[216] I think of how love intrinsically embeds itself in the creation of a politicized, disabled, queer of color beauty politic. We do not have to find ourselves and our beauties alone; our communities can become our doulas.

––––––––

During her/their performance in *Birthing, Dying, Becoming Crip Wisdom*, Leah Lakshmi Piepzna-Samarasinha sits and moves back and forth on a rocking chair. In "Crip Magic Spells" she/they are our crip fairy god-mother and she/they appear on stage with incantations of survival, with what she/they call a "cheat sheet" for our crip futures. Leah's first lesson to us is that we must remember the persistence of our beauty and magic as we crip our way through the ableism of this world:

This is not in any pamphlet they send you home from the hospital with.
This is operating instructions. I mean to save your life with what I was

taught in the secret guild of other sickos, with what I learned the hard way. Dear baby crip, it's not all bad news. This is the magic skill I'm calling into existence. … I know it's going to take at least ten years for you to not, maybe, sort of hate yourself, but I invoke that you will. This is a magic spell because we write the future with our bodies every day. … you will gain a wild pack of crip fam … I invoke that you will drool, type, stim and shake with joy. You will move as slow and weird as you want, and others will roll and limp with you in a wild pack of slowness.

Leah invokes crip beauty as accompaniment: we will live and learn about ourselves in community. We will live in a time and in a place

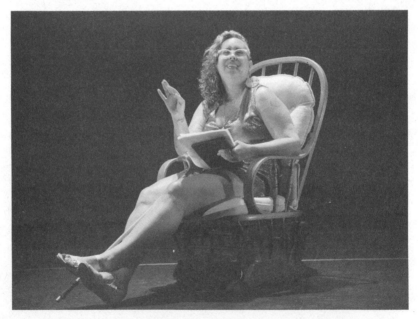

Leah Lakshmi Piepzna-Samarasinha in "Crip Magic Spells", 2016. *Birthing, Dying, Becoming Crip Wisdom*, ODC Theater. Photo by Richard Downing, courtesy of Sins Invalid.

surrounded by the love conjurings of our crip elders and ancestors. We will live an infusion of hurt, beauty, and messy joy because, when we find our crip kin, we will not have to do it alone.

Patty expands on the construction of beauty as a communal lesson when she/they address the ways our bodyminds have been forcefully distanced from beauty: "I think we must decolonize ourselves, play large, know our fabulousness, our worth, our power in the face of being told that our beauty could not be. When I say beauty, I mean a beauty based in our integrity, our lineages, our aesthetics ... a beauty that radiates from our hearts, not from symmetrical bone structure."[217]

Beauty as lineage is communal labor; it is love labor. For Patty, and for Sins Invalid, it aids in the creation of a liberated culture.[218] All of their framings of queering, cripping, and decolonizing beauty urge us to push back and resist the restriction of beauty norms that eradicate our intrinsic and communal potential and knowledge. To ensure the liberation and survival of all our bodyminds, we must collectively cocreate new realities and new futures where our disabled, queer of color bodyminds can practice ways to liberate beauty. Above all, we must remember that our communities can be curative, that we are surrounded by crip fairy godmothers and, as Leah says, "a wild pack of crip fam."

In striving to birth ourselves, in striving to restore our bodyminds as the resilient beings that we are, we need to center beauty. We need to speak about beauty as liberation, as a radically cripped, queered, and decolonized offering. We also need to imagine what this kind of refashioning looks like so that we know how to access it and apply it to our own lives. In response to our wonderings and curiosities, Sins Invalid offers us examples of what it means to have an unshamed claim to beauty that is accessible, inclusive, and loving; they offer us crip beauty as a way home.

CHAPTER 10

Manifesting Our Collective Futures

Revolutions begin with rest,[219] with time to think, feel, and create our way into dreaming new realities. Sins Invalid comes from this place, from the star stuff of crip dreams and crip aspirations. With our disabled, queer of color dreams, our hearts and guts speak to us in rest; they tell us that there are ways to live, love, and thrive without exhaustion. Our hearts and guts tell us that now is the time to create crip-centric liberated zones and to live and enact Disability Justice organizing. We may not survive without it.

Dreaming gives us the opportunity to slow down and practice what Tricia Hersey, Nap Bishop and founder of the Nap Ministry, calls the anti-capitalist, anti-racist, anti-ableist magic of napping. Tricia urges that rest is "a spiritual practice. Rest is productive;"[220] rest is where we imagine. Resting and dreaming, in this context, are not passive. They are full of electric possibility. For Tricia, to rest is to create enough space to pause and reflect. In reflection, rest and the dreaming that comes from this transformative place have the potential to rebel, to push back, and to resist. Rest, as Tricia writes, is activism, a politicized, agentic act. During an interview with journalist Maya Kroth, Tricia says that naps take us beyond the act of sleeping: "This is not just about naps … It's about trying to disrupt and dismantle a toxic system that says you are not enough."[221] In this new framing, naps offer us moments where we can create the liberatory realities we have been waiting for. When the most disempowered of us slows down enough to rest, enough to nap, we harness the energy to enact revolutionary shifts or, as Tricia says, to dismantle the toxic oppressions that hold our bodyminds in passive distraction. Removing guilt and shame from rest is how we will move ourselves in wholeness and sustainability.[222]

I find generative possibility here between Tricia's call for naps and Leah Lakshmi Piepzna-Samarasinha's offering that when disabled, queer of color communities dream, they create revolution. In her/their essay "Cripping the Apocalypse: Some of My Wild Disability Justice Dreams," Leah offers readers this incantation: "Sick and disabled and neurodivergent folks aren't supposed to dream, especially if we are queer and Black or Brown—we're just supposed to be grateful the 'normals' let us live. But I am the product of some wild disabled Black and Brown queer revolutionary dreaming."[223] Dreaming disabled, queer of color dreams creates portals, openings where we can enter to create change. The intersection of slowing down and dreaming is where our disabled, queer of color futures come from. Disabled, queer of color community dreamed Disability Justice to strategize our collective liberation. This is also where Sins Invalid came from: a crip love that dreamed open a revolutionary future for all our bodyminds.

"Inhale the dust of possibility. Exhale dreams."

To dream disabled, queer of color futures is a profound and bountiful act, particularly since time does not function the same for all of us. Its linear progression restricts and does not honor our queer bodyminds or our disabled bodies.[224] Alison Kafer writes that "curative time" particularly limits and suspends the futures of disabled bodyminds.[225] As we live governed by nondisabled supremacy, a crip future without a cure is unimaginable, and for Alison, "*we* need to imagine crip futures because disabled people are continually being written out of the future, rendered as a sign of the future no one wants ... We must begin to anticipate presents and to imagine futures that include all of us."[226] This, as mediated through their Disability Justice politics, is precisely where Sins Invalid directs us. The performance project gives us a tangible place where we can witness our crip, queer, decolonial histories, our present, and our futures.

Birthing, Dying, Becoming Crip Wisdom directly explores what our future making could look like. I understood this performance as an answer to a call: how do we manifest *us* and *we* in a liberatory and generative future? How can we, in our present moment, even imagine such a place? I think here of future makers such as James Baldwin, Alexis Pauline Gumbs, Kay Ulanday Barrett, Marsha P. Johnson, Sylvia Rivera, and Grace Lee Boggs, who speak to the importance of *us* and *we* in the creation of futures. *Us* and *we* are how we move toward creating something liberatory and necessary from the margins. It is how we create liberated zones, and, most critically, it is how we move toward thriving. This important work cannot happen, however, until we pause, rest, and dream. We cannot create the world without the anti-capitalist act of

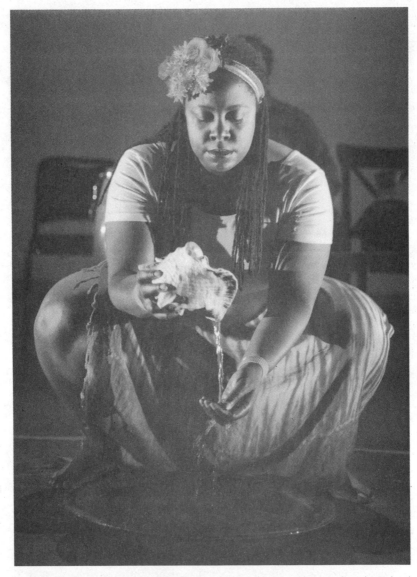

India Harville, 2016. *Birthing, Dying, Becoming Crip Wisdom*, ODC Theater. Photo by Richard Downing, courtesy of Sins Invalid.

slowing down and taking stock of what no longer serves us. We cannot challenge and recreate oppression if we are exhausted and overworked.[227]

The beginning of *Birthing, Dying, Becoming Crip Wisdom* invites us to reflect and to create our disabled, queer of color futures. A group of Haitian drummers dressed in white walk through the audience and toward the stage. As they move, we hear the shaking of gourds, the pounding of drums, and the guttural sounds of a conch shell; they are opening a space of invitation. India Harville appears onstage. She is surrounded by a blue light, and she begins to move like water as the invocation continues overhead: "It is not an accident that we are gathered here. Each one of us was summoned to this place, to this moment, to be imaginers. The earth is a beautiful crip grandmother trembling with sickness, singing through her pain, swaying her mountainous hips, calling us here … Inhale, exhale. Inhale the dust of possibility. Exhale dreams."

India's body encourages us to reflect and to awaken, to view ourselves as dreamers who can shift, create, and implement change-making. Our lives are revolution, and we have within our bodyminds the courageous power to establish change. To position us, the disabled, queer of color many, as creators of our future centers that we indeed *have* futures: more than a longing, our futures are a tangible reality.

———

"The work of supporting people rebirthing themselves as disabled or more disabled has a name. We are doulas."

Although the reminder and refrain that we are creators of our own futures energizes and invigorates me, it also leaves me with questions. How do we begin to do this work? Even after all the internal adjustments and empowered transformations take place, how do we begin manifesting a future for all our bodyminds? The first answer to this question comes from crip ancestor Stacey Milbern. During episode six of the *Disability Visibility Podcast*, Alice Wong interviewed Stacey and Leah about the labor and work of disabled queer femmes of color. In particular, Stacey spoke about crip doulas: "The work of supporting people rebirthing themselves as disabled or more disabled has a name. We are doulas. Crip mentorship/coaching/modeling at its best is disability doulaship. The fact that society doesn't even have language to describe this transition speaks to the ableism and isolation people with disabilities face in figuring out how to be in their bodyminds and in this ableist world."[228]

Amid nondisabled supremacy, its messages, and its restrictions, a crip doula is a supportive guide. Crip doulas stress that we do not grow into our present or our futures on our own; we move into these places with the love and mentorship of our community. Together, we rebirth ourselves into our disabilities or into our shifting disabled bodyminds. We do this work with celebration and with struggle, but we never journey alone.[229] Crip doulaship centers communal appreciation and acknowledgment, and it is, as Stacey argues, necessary for our "survival and resilience."[230]

Sins Invalid exists for so many of us as our crip doulas, as a network of support, recognition, and love reminding us that we are deserving; we have *always* been deserving. The performance project extends crip doulaship past the individual and anticipates Disability Justice and communal artmaking as guide, as what Stacey calls "crip intervention." During a conversation with Stacey about crip doulas, Leah reflects that doulas bring us "a huge paradigm shift—the view coming into disability identity as a birth, not a death, which is how the transition(s) are seen by ableist culture."[231] Sins Invalid's Disability Justice organizing, their performances, workshops, trainings, and online content provide us with the guidebook we need to rebirth ourselves into our power and into our persistence. We create ourselves outside of ableism as our vulnerable, adventurous, soft, and growing selves. In this new place of rebirthing, we can live in a future that honors the legacies of our ancestors of color, our queer, gender nonconforming, trans ancestors, our disabled, chronically ill, and Mad knowledge makers.

Sins Invalid's 2016 performance aided all of us toward crip rebirth. With its focus on crip wisdom and knowledge sharing, it gave us strategies for our continued survival during a time of uncertainty. Leah's performance, "Crip Magic Spells," became for me a manifestation of crip doulaship: we are not in this alone. Standing, cane in hand, Leah begins:

> Beautiful baby crip. I come to you in your dreams. There is so much no one is going to tell you, for a while. Please don't die … no one is telling you that disability is magic, that crips are magicians, that is so very important that you live …. We are waiting for you. We are going to be what saves your life. We are here to tell you how we do it, how keep doing it. We flourish the swords and wands of this artful way to live …. There is no such thing as not disabled enough …. There is no such thing as being

too disabled to live in this world .... But every day is a new chance to practice your magic.

The crip doula, for Leah, embodies intergenerational knowledges: all the messy realizations, the painful knowings, and the spells that will propel us, the disabled many, through nondisabled supremacy, through ableism, through it all toward crip survival and future making. Their insistence on the word "we" returns me to Stacey's original crafting of crip doulas as community workers. In "Crip Magic Spells," Leah as crip doula gives us a survivor guide so that we can live and manifest a disabled, queer of color future that is uniquely our own, a future that continues a legacy of endurance and crip love.

"Crip Magic Spells" moves us toward crip rebirth, toward connectivity and community; we are given survival tools for a world regulated by nondisabled supremacy, by racism, and by cis-heteropatriarchy. The truths Leah urges us toward are profound: we deserve, we are enough, and we are valid in our mess and in our needs. For Leah, and by extension Sins Invalid, survival in community is how we will endure, how we grow resilient and true. We thrive because we teach one another how to resource share and how to hack ableism. We thrive because we impart the wisdom we have struggled to gather. As a communal crip doula, Sins Invalid's Disability Justice and artmaking practices move our body-minds toward persistence.

> "We know now, and I think most people
> knew then, but maybe were scared to claim,
> that our dear, sweet, lovable, sexy, hardworking,
> soft, hard bodies are never problems.
> We are never problems."

As a presenter during Movement Generation's Course Correction webinar, "Decolonize the Future," Patty joined from the year 2050 to report on the progress that Disability Justice organizers had made. She/they began by naming that in the future, our needs are no longer met with shame. Our needs are addressed in public with what Patty calls support teams: "[there are] amazing support teams that are on every corner so wherever we go we can get childcare, we can be assisted to eat, we can take a shit, we can take a nap."[232] In the future, we do not need to ask that our needs be met in hushed, whispered tones. The future is radically interdependent. In this new place, we live in community with an entire social body who also needs, who also pauses for assistance, who also asks for exactly what they need when they need it. In the future, crip-centric liberated zones are no longer isolated to specific places, venues, or events; they are simply everywhere.

Patty shares that in this revolutionary crip future, organizers understand that to live and create change, we must work in connection both with ourselves and with one another. In reflection, she/they says: "Back then folks were trying to control their bodies, and the land, and the sky, and time. People were still thinking that the world around them was separate from their bodies, and their bodies were separate from their psyches ...."

We have done a lot of work to align ourselves in our wholeness and that means going through our ancestors' trauma and working with healers now to address all the epigenetic changes that have occurred."[233]

In the future we organize without exclusion. In wholeness and in alignment with our bodyminds, our histories, and with the understanding that our identities intersect, we coordinate for a liberation that is genuine in its acknowledgement of our bodymind needs. We, in community, evolve.

To emerge from this collective place of organizing requires that we understand our bodyminds not as problems but as openings, as entry points to our shared humanity. This was, for me, one of the ripest offerings from Patty's future. She/they began by saying, "We know now, and I think people knew then but were maybe scared to claim, that our dear, sweet, lovable, sexy, hardworking, soft, hard bodies are never problems. We are never problems."[234] This statement conjures possibility. It is a communal love letter from Disability Justice organizers in 2050 to all of us. It is the loving insistence that we are enough.

For Patty, our disabled, queer of color bodyminds are not defects, errors, or in need of revision; rather, the systems around us are in need of change: "What's a problem is a social and economic system that excludes people like us ... We have always been here. Disabled, Black, Indigenous people of color, queer, trans, gender nonbinary, disabled people have always been here because we are a beautiful part of humanity, a very natural part of what it means to be on the planet."[235]

What Patty brings us from the future is an awakening on the largest scale. There is nothing inherently wrong with us; there is, however, something wrong with the systems of oppression that systemically regulate us. We are beautiful and necessary in all our cripness, in all our color, in our queerness, in our gender nonconformity and transness. We are necessary just as we are.

Patty's words leave me with an eagerly felt promise: collective liberation for all our bodyminds *comes*; with our collective liberation and care work, it comes. Crip-centric liberated zones and all their glorious, accessible gifts come. Growth and learning in slowness, in sustainability comes, and we get there with our collective love and labor. Our disabled, queer of color future is a manifestation and affirmation of abundance.

Why All This Matters

"We are powerful because we have survived."

—AUDRE LORDE

In describing Sins Invalid, I find myself returning, again and again, to the idea of an invitation: Patty, Leroy, and the entire Sins Invalid community are seedlings that together ask that we create something magnetic out of all the chaos and oppression because, in the end, empowered with our crip, queer, decolonial lineage, we are the only ones who can.

Dear reader: it is time for us to gather and attune ourselves to communal learning. We need to justice-seek our way toward repair; our lives depend on it. Since they began their work in 2006, Sins Invalid has taught us that revolution is not a fleeting or solely aspirational thing; rather, it is as Sammie Ablaza Wills suggests, a practice: "Revolution is not a moment. It is a practice. It is a culture of making mistakes, of transforming harm, of celebrating joy." In our disabled, queer of color communities, so much of our lineage calls on the recovery of histories and stories. This, for me, has everything to do with love and with the radical care of our coalitional work. For Sins Invalid, this crip lineage is a gathered, tended-to thing. It comes from communal restlessness, a knowing that disabled, queer of color knowledge is always collective, cocreated medicine for our survival.

———————

Patty and Leroy's initial dinner conversation brought with it the affirmation that disabled bodyminds have the right to pleasure, to the sensual, to the decadent, and to the beautiful. Disabled, queer of color bodyminds deserve futurity. They deserve to fuck, to masturbate, to soak in bodies of water, to adorn themselves in glitter, petals, and honey. At the same time, their gut knowledge offers audiences spaces of possibility that are not devoid of risk. To present Black, queer, disabled lovers on stage, a Latina's wheelchair striptease, or kinky powerplay between a transmasculine poet and a Maori disabled wheelchair user is not without risk. In centering the transformative potential of disabled, queer, transgender, and gender nonconforming performers of color onstage, and in developing uniquely crip cultures of sexuality and beauty, Sins Invalid politicizes what our bodyminds are *allowed* to do.

In this new culture of permission, the performance project encourages us to imagine and then declare our bodymind lessons and journeys as proof that we, despite it all, are still here. We are storytellers. We are protest. We are crip kinship networks vast, bold, and soft. With their Disability Justice–led practice for revolution, we are given a map leading us through stereotype and oppression so that we can begin to imagine our bodyminds as the unapologetic, fabulous change-makers they are.

———————

Cripping the Future

Throughout writing this book, I have found myself returning to Sins Invalid's crip-centric liberated zones. I have written about what they do and why they are so necessary, but I have struggled to describe what they feel like. As I finished reading Alice Wong's anthology *Disability Visibility: First-Person Stories from the Twenty-First Century*, I read s.e. smith's (they/them) chapter, "The Beauty of Spaces Created for and by Disabled People." In describing what shared "crip spaces" offer, they provided me with the language I had been searching for:

> The first *social* setting where you come to the giddy understanding that this is a place for disabled people is a momentous one, and one worth lingering over. I cannot remember the first time it happened to me—perhaps a house party in San Francisco or an art show or a meeting of friends at a café. The experiences blend together, creating a sense of crip space, a communal belonging, a deep *rightness*, that comes from not having to justify your existence. They are resting points, even as they can be energizing and exhilarating.[236]

I read and reread s.e.'s descriptors of crip space: "a communal belonging," "a deep *rightness*," a "giddy" place. A crip space is, as they tell us, both a place of rest and of exhilaration; it is a feeling place of communal appreciation. This "deep *rightness*" is what our disabled, queer of color bodyminds crave. Crip-centric liberated zones and their multidirectional love practices produce for us and with us these places of *rightness*. In love, we search for a rightness, a cozy gut feeling where we can grow and support each other in wholeness. A cozy gut feeling becomes an assemblage of recognition and validation, a distinct awareness that our disabled bodyminds are worthy of celebration, life, and futurity; it is a feeling that affirms all of us who are *also*: *also* trans, queer, and gender non-conforming; *also* houseless, undocumented, and incarcerated; *also* impoverished, and under- or unemployed disabled bodyminds; and *also* people of color who are trying to survive. It is restorative to embrace and invite all of us who are *also* into the future, so that we can collectively persist in our defiant dreams of disabled, queer of color worlds.

Sins Invalid brings out in us giddy *rightness* through the crip-centric strategies of storytelling and artmaking, Disability Justice–based education, and online crip kinship networks. There is a newness, a surprise, and perhaps an abrupt shock when we learn that we can relish in our disabled, queer of color community and the justice centered futures we have and will continue to create. There is elation and wonderment when we gather together and we can watch—in all the different ways watching happens—beauty and sensuality turned into verbs, into the resistance tools that we can use to dismantle nondisabled supremacy and all the toxicity that it collides and works with. Perhaps this is the biggest gift Sins Invalid gives us: the vocabulary, guidance, and methods for a social and political revolution that fearlessly centers the knowledge production of disabled, queer of color communities.

––––––––

During one of our final conversations, I asked Patty and Nomy to share their hopes for the performance project. Holding on to Disability Justice's urging that the future is the "yet-to-be,"[237] what changes do they plan to enact? What transformations? Because the medical industrial complex—and its ableism, racism, cis-heteropatriarchy, capitalism, and fat phobia—does not create networks of justice, care, or wellness for all our bodyminds, Sins Invalid intends to create retirement and healthcare funds for their crip elders. They are also laying the groundwork for Sins University, a place where community can gather to learn from the performance project's unique synthesis of Disability Justice movement and organizational building work and artmaking.

To continue extending their reach and access, in 2020 they launched *Into the Crip Universe: Cripping the Anthropocene*, a new podcast series hosted by Rafi Ruffino Darrow; season one dedicates itself to the current climate crises and each subsequent season will unpack another theme through conversations with artist-activists and educators. This is, I think, what crip dreaming cultivates: a constant, slow, intentional, and determined creation of new ways to sustain and empower us, new ways to move us toward revolution.

You Are Invited

Dear giddy dream maker, dear future seeker, dear crip kin: what direction will *your* yet-to-be map take you? How will you support your bodymind and the bodyminds of others as you embark on this journey? What elements are a necessity in your expression of bodymind reclamation, recognition, and storytelling? How will you integrate Disability Justice into the practices of your everyday living and organizing? You play an active part in creating crip-centric liberated zones and microcultures full of love. *You* do that. Pause to ask yourself what your microculture looks like. What does it feel like? How does it nourish you? How can you create a path of interconnection between your place of flourishing and the next person's? What are the gifts only *you* can bring?

I end with these questions and offer them to you as starting points. They are the fledgling stuff that has created space for all of this disabled, queer of color changemaking. What other questions and ponderings does Sins Invalid motivate you toward? Imagine yourself sitting alongside them: what cripped out futures do you want to dream up, together? May you, dear one, write the next book, and the next, as we continue to move together toward our collective bodymind liberation.

NOTES

[1] As the shortened version of the derogatory slur "cripple," crip has been reappropriated by some in the disability community and is now being used as a politicized term of empowerment. Some folks of color spell it with a "k": krip. Its reclamation has been likened to the word "queer." One pitfall of the term as identified by Alison Kafer (2013), however, is that crip often only refers to physical disabilities and can be limiting in this way.

[2] The capitalization of Mad signals the work and activism of Mad activists and Mad Studies scholars who argue that we need to problematize the stigmatic and negative connotations of madness. I will capitalize the word Mad throughout the book to honor this work; I also capitalize Mad as it is an identity within which I am located.

[3] The bodymind is a term of unification suggesting that our bodies and our minds never engage in isolation from one another. This concept has Indigenous roots. For more information, explore *Sharing Breath: Embodied Learning and Decolonization*, edited by Sheila Batacharya and Yuk-Lin Renita Wong.

[4] Audism is a system of discrimination and prejudice particularly directed against those belonging to the Deaf or hard of hearing community.

[5] The phrase "disabled, queer of color bodymind" is going to be used throughout the book as shorthand. It is a phrase that acknowledges Sins Invalid's intersection of artist-activists who are disabled, chronically ill, and/or Mad, who are queer, gender nonconforming, and/or trans, and who are people of color. When necessary for clarity, I will be more specific about the communities I am discussing.

[6] Road, Cristy C., *Next World Tarot* (Croad Core Art).

[7] There are many intersecting oppressions that relegate our disabled lives. For consistency, I will focus on ableism, racism, and cis-heteropatriarchy. Although this list is abbreviated, it most closely addresses what Sins Invalid seeks to revise. When necessary for clarity, I will be more specific about the systems of oppression I am exploring.

[8] Disability Studies scholars like Alison Kafer (2013), Margaret Price (2016), and Ellen Samuels (2017) have written about crip time as a shifting of normative time: "rather than bend disabled bodies and minds to meet the clock, crip time bends the clock to meet disabled bodies and minds" (Kafer, 2013, 27). To work in crip time is to work at the pace that honors the needs and capacities of our disabled, Mad, chronically ill bodyminds.

9 For more information on the Black Lives Matter protests that took place in the summer of 2020, including statistics and maps, visit nytimes.com/interactive/2020/07/03/us/george -floyd-protests-crowd-size.html

10 Lewis, Talila, *Resistance and Hope: Crip Wisdom for the People*.

11 Berne, Patty, Skype interview, April 2018.

12 Disability historian Paul Longmore identifies that the first wave of the Disability Rights Movement began in the 1930s and carried into the 1990s. Disability Justice activists identify that the second wave of the movement began in 2005 with the creation of Disability Justice.

13 Miles, Nishida, and Forber-Pratt 2017; Lewis 2019; O'Toole 2019; Berne 2015; Bell 2011.

14 Thompson, Vilissa, "Appropriation in the Disability Community: We Are Our Own Worst Enemy."

15 Wong, Alice, "Not a Unicorn: Finding Communities Within a Community."

16 The mainstream feminist and the mainstream LGBTQIA+ movements have also struggled with acknowledging, including, and honoring the diversity in their communities.

17 The term people of color began with the labor and organizing of Black women during the 1977 National Women's Conference, and it is a "solidarity definition," a "political designation" (Loretta Ross, 2011). I am using the phrase people of color (POC) as opposed to Black, Indigenous, People of Color (BIPOC), aware that both acronyms cause a level of harm and erasure. No single acronym can acknowledge the lived reality of our diverse identities (Sarmistha Talukdar, 2021); however, POC aligns more closely with politics rather than racialized identities.

18 Piepzna-Samarasinha, Leah Lakshmi, *Care Work: Dreaming Disability Justice*.

19 Lorde, Audre, "Learning from the 60s."

20 Sins Invalid, *Skin, Tooth, and Bone—The Basis of Our Movement Is Our People*, 20.

21 Lewis, Talila A., "Ableism 2020: An Updated Definition."

22 hooks, bell, *Yearning: Race, Gender, and Cultural Politics*.

23 Lamm, Nomy, "This Is Disability Justice."

24 Sins Invalid, *Skin, Tooth, and Bone*.

[25] Berne, Patty. "Disability Justice—A Working Draft by Patty Berne."

[26] Deaf with a capital D indicates an honoring of Deaf identity, culture, language, and community. Lowercase-d deaf, on the other hand, only references the physicality of hearing loss.

[27] Ahmed, Sara, *Living a Feminist Life*, 81.

[28] Ahmed, Sara, *Living a Feminist Life*, 15–16.

[29] Krip, instead of crip, is an intentional modification in spelling that alludes to the intersection of race and disability. Some disabled people of color use this spelling to address the politicization of their intersectional identities.

[30] Berne, Patty and Jamal T. Lewis et al., "'Beauty Always Recognizes Itself': A Roundtable on Sins Invalid," 202.

[31] Berne et al., "Sins Invalid: Disability, Dancing, and Claiming Beauty," 203.

[32] Ugly laws existed during the nineteenth and twentieth centuries. As an ableist and classist legislation, it outlawed people who were "diseased, maimed, mutilated, or in any way deformed, so as to be an unsightly or disgusting object" (Chicago City Code 1881). For information about the ugly laws and their impact, explore Susan M. Schweik's 2009 book, *The Ugly Laws: Disability in Public.*

[33] Kuttner, Paul, "An Interview with Sins Invalid."

[34] Berne, et al., "Sins Invalid: Disability, Dancing, and Claiming Beauty," 204.

[35] Sins Invalid, *Skin, Tooth, and Bone*, 23.

[36] Berne, Patty, personal interview, 2014.

[37] Currently, Todd Herman and Amanda Coslor are artistic advisors and have left the core organizational structure of Sins Invalid. Patty is the executive and artistic director and Nomy Lamm is the creative director. The performance project is also supported by a program team, including interns and a developmental director that works on fiscal management and fundraising. Sins Invalid is currently in the process of hiring an administrative and development associate to help with the daily organizational needs of the performance project.

[38] Anzaldúa, *Light in the Dark/Luz en lo Oscuro*, 44.

[39] Anzaldúa, *Light in the Dark/Luz en lo Oscuro*, 40.

[40] Taylor, Sonya Renee, *The Body Is Not an Apology*, 6.

[41] Taylor, *The Body Is Not an Apology*, 10.

[42] Berne, Patty, personal interview. 2018.

[43] Sins Invalid's mission statement includes a diverse and expansive definition of disability: "We define disability broadly to include people with physical impairments, people who belong to a sensory minority, people with emotional disabilities, people with cognitive challenges, and those with chronic/severe illness. We understand the experience of disability to occur within any and all walks of life, with deeply felt connections to all communities impacted by the medicalization of their bodies, including trans, gender variant and intersex people, and others whose bodies do not conform to culture(s)' notions of 'normal' or 'functional.'" They apply this definition to the performers they support as well as the content they produce.

[44] Berne, Patty, personal interview, 2014.

[45] Sins Invalid, *Skin, Tooth, and Bone*, 16.

[46] When I think of the disposability of disabled, queer of color communities, I am thinking of the many institutional ways these communities are disenfranchised and under- or unemployed. I am thinking of police brutality, systemic violence, and the prison industrial complex.

[47] Berne, Patty, "Sins Invalid: Disability, Dancing, and Claiming Beauty," 207.

[48] Pernick, Martin S., "The Body and Physical Difference," 90.

[49] Kuttner, Paul, "An Interview with Sins Invalid."

[50] Devlieger, Patrick J., "Generating a Cultural Model of Disability," 8.

[51] Kuttner, Paul, "An Interview with Sins Invalid."

[52] A killjoy is someone who, as Sara Ahmed writes in *Living a Feminist Life*, "'spoils' the happiness of otherness; she is a spoilsport because she refuses to convene, to assemble, or to meet up over happiness. In the thick sociality of everyday spaces, feminists are thus attributed as the origin of the bad feeling, as the ones who ruin the atmosphere."

[53] Ahmed, *Living a Feminist Life*, 84.

[54] Disabled activist and comedian Stella Young developed the term "inspiration porn" in 2012. Inspiration porn argues that our ableist culture only portrays disabled bodyminds in inspirational ways, reducing them to one-dimensional objects.

[55] Sins Invalid, *Skin, Tooth, and Bone*, 26.

[56] Sins Invalid, *Skin, Tooth, and Bone*, 26. The phrase "leaves no bodymind behind" is a contribution from Sins Invalid member and Disability Justice organizer Lezlie Frye.

[57] Mingus, Mia, "Access Intimacy: The Missing Link."

[58] Mingus, "Access Intimacy: The Missing Link."

[59] Sins Invalid, *Skin, Tooth, and Bone*, 26.

[60] Asher, Nina, "Writing Home/Decolonizing Text(s)," 2.

[61] Frantz Fanon's (1967) work in his seminal text, *Black Skin, White Masks*, informs Nina Asher's focus on disembodiment and dislocation.

[62] Fanon, Frantz 1967; Said, Edward 1978.

[63] Asher, Nina 2009; Fanon, Frantz 1967; hooks, bell 1990; Trinh, Thi Minh-Ha 1989.

[64] The 2015 visual art exhibit and performance *Disability Liberated* was created in response to the 2014 anthology *Disability Incarcerated: Imprisonment and Disability in the United States and Canada*.

[65] Washington, Harriet A., *Medical Apartheid: The Dark History of Medical Experimentation on Black Americans from Colonial Times to the Present*, 26.

[66] Berne, Patty, personal interview, 2018.

[67] Berne et al., "Sins Invalid: Disability, Dancing, and Claiming Beauty," 420.

[68] Sins Invalid, "Behind the Scenes with the Performers of Disability Liberated."

[69] Lakshmi, Leah Piepzna-Samarasinha, personal interview, 2016.

[70] "Witness," in *Lexico*.

[71] Berne, personal interview, 2014.

[72] Leah Lakshmi Piepzna-Samarasinha first learned of mutual aid in the works of writer Ursula K. Le Guin, geographer Peter Kropotkin, and queer feminists and anarchists.

[73] Piepzna-Samarasinha, *Care Work*, 41.

[74] Piepzna-Samarasinha, *Care Work*, 41–42.

[75] Black, Rebel Sidney, "Pod Mapping for Mutual Aid," March 9, 2020.

[76] Stryker, Kitty, "Collective Care Is Our Best Weapon against COVID-19."

[77] Stimulus sharing platforms such as sharemycheck.org have aided in the dispersal of stimulus checks, as have individual campaigns on social media platforms such as Twitter and Instagram.

[78] New York, in particular, has created a map of free community refrigerators and pantries that are available to the public. The UK also uses this format; their community refrigerators and pantries follow models developed in Germany and Spain.

[79] Beyond local and national mutual aid maps, community members can access a global interactive mutual aid map by visiting covidmutualaid.org/local-groups/.

[80] Similar to the applications and stretching of subtext that "queering" as a verb invites, disability performance scholar and artist Carrie Sandahl suggests that cripping carries a similar resonance. She writes that cripping "spins mainstream representations or practices to reveal able-bodied assumptions." Cripping is a troubling, a door opening to invite us toward challenging what is normal and what we assume is defective.

[81] Sins Invalid, "Show Your Cripself That You Are Loved."

[82] Sins Invalid, "Show Your Cripself That You Are Loved."

[83] Sins Invalid, "Show Your Cripself That You Are Loved."

[84] hooks, bell, *All About Love*, xix.

[85] hooks, *All About Love*, xix.

[86] hooks, bell, *Outlaw Culture: Resisting Representation*.

[87] hooks, *Outlaw Culture*, 249.

[88] hooks, *Outlaw Culture*, 248.

[89] *What, How, and Why Not*.

[90] Sins Invalid, *Skin, Tooth, and Bone*, 8.

[91] Although Arthur W. Frank does not use the more contemporary term bodymind in his discussion of storytelling through the body, I have added it here to stay consistent with my use of language.

[92] Frank, Arthur W., *The Wounded Storyteller*, 2.

[93] Berne et al., "'Beauty Always Recognizes Itself,'" 243.

[94] Movement Generation Justice & Ecology Project is led by communities of color and low-income communities whose mission is to bring "liberation and restoration of land, labor, and culture" back into these notoriously neglected and disenfranchised communities. Movement Generation's 2020 *Course Correction* is an online course series aiming to address the structural inequalities, solutions, and strategies surrounding the COVID-19 pandemic. For more information, visit movementgeneration.org.

[95] Frank, Arthur W., *The Wounded Storyteller*, 2.

[96] Berne, personal interview, 2014.

[97] Frank, Arthur W., *The Wounded Storyteller*, xii.

[98] Taylor, Sonya Renee, *The Body Is Not an Apology*, 12.

[99] Moore, Leroy F., personal narrative, April 2016.

[100] Anzaldúa, Gloria, *Borderlands/La Frontera: The New Mestiza*, 75.

[101] Anzaldúa, *Borderlands/La Frontera*, 75.

[102] Although Gloria Anzaldúa never self-identified as having a disability, I call her forward here as one of my crip elders. In her posthumously published book *Light in the Dark/Luz en lo Oscuro*, she wrote, for example, about how her hormonal imbalance, her diabetes, and her body pain sculpted how she wrote and theorized.

[103] Anzaldúa, *Borderlands/La Frontera*, 81.

[104] *Creating Art as Resistance to Ableism.*

[105] *Creating Art as Resistance to Ableism.*

[106] *Creating Art as Resistance to Ableism.*

[107] Irani, Kayhan, "Introduction," 5.

[108] Solórzano, Daniel G., and Tara J. Yosso, "Critical Race Methodology," 28.

[109] Solórzano and Yosso, "Critical Race Methodology," 29.

[110] Solórzano and Yosso, "Critical Race Methodology," 31.

[111] Irani, Kayhan, "Introduction," 6.

[112] Sins Invalid, *Skin, Tooth, and Bone*, 26.

[113] Paul K. Longmore Institute on Disability, "Alice Wong Longmore Lecture with Video and Transcript: 'Storytelling as Activism: The Politics of Disability Visibility.'"

[114] Berne, personal interview, April 2016.

[115] Steinberg, David, "Sins Invalid: An Unshamed Look at Sex, Beauty, and Disability

[116] Dufour, Kirsten, "Art as Activism, Activism as Art," 157.

[117] Barndt, Deborah, *Wild Fire: Art as Activism.*

[118] Barndt, *Wild Fire*, 18.

[119] Kuttner, Paul, "An Interview with Sins Invalid."

[120] Kuttner, Paul, "An Interview with Sins Invalid."

[121] Sins Invalid, *Skin, Tooth, and Bone*, 24–25.

[122] Not everyone experiences time linearly. It can be queered (Keeling 2019; Halberstam 2005; Edelman 2004), cripped (Samuels 2017; Kafer 2013), and informed by communities of color ("ColoredPeopleTime") (Keeling 2019).

[123] Price, Margaret, *Mad at School*, 62.

[124] Kafer, Alison, *Feminist, Queer, Crip*, 27.

[125] Samuels, Ellen, "Six Ways of Looking at Crip Time."

[126] Although disability studies scholars have written about the benefits and liberatory aspects of crip time (Kafer 2013; Price 2011), it is important to note that Ellen Samuels (2017) addresses the isolation and the pitfalls of crip time.

[127] Crutchfield, Susan and Marcy Epstein, *Points of Contact: Disability, Art, and Culture.*

[128] Sutherland, Allan, "Disability Arts, Disability Politics."

[129] "*Disability Visibility Project*: Mia Mingus, Part 3."

[130] "*Disability Visibility Project*: Mia Mingus, Part 3."

[131] Sins Invalid, *Skin, Tooth, and Bone*, 26.

[132] "Everyday Abolition/Abolition Everyday Interview with Leroy Moore."

[133] Sins Invalid, *Skin, Tooth, and Bone*, 5.

[134] Kunimoto, Ai, , Shotaro Kinoshita, and Tsumki Nakamura, "'I Had to Do It for Society': Conversations with Accused Japan Care Home Mass Murderer."

[135] Eugenics in Japan did not end until 1996, when the country passed the Eugenics Protection Law to abolish the sterilization of the disability community. Since eugenics was enacted in 1948, approximately 25,000 people were sterilized, many without their consent. For more information, visit japantimes.co.jp/opinion/2020/02/13/editorials/coming-terms-whats-behind-sagamihara-killings/.

[136] It is necessary that we view Satoshi Uematsu's story through an intersectional lens. What larger conversations does this single incident urge us toward? What is Japan's cultural attitude toward disabilities? Satoshi was hospitalized and diagnosed with what the medical industrial complex names a delusional disorder but left treatment before committing the murders. What local/global conversations does this invite in regard to mental health care?

[137] Takenaka, Kiyoshi, "Japanese Man Pleads Not Guilty."

[138] The language of crip community as doula comes from Staccy Milbern and a conversation she had with Alice Wong and Leah Lakshmi Piepzna-Samarasinha in 2017 on the *Disability Visibility Podcast* (disabilityvisibllityproject.com/2017/10/22/ep-6-labor-care-work-and-disabled-queer-femmes/).

[139] KHOU Staff, "Last Dance: More than 1,000 People Turn Out for Dying Teen's Prom."

[140] Sins Invalid, *Skin, Tooth, and Bone*, 12.

[141] Kafer, Alison, *Feminist, Queer, Crip*, 9.

[142] Performance artist and scholar Petra Kuppers (2014) has specified that although some experiences are embodied, because the body informs the mind and the mind informs the body, when we discuss experiences, we need to hold space for the embodied and the enminded. I use her language of the embodied/enminded to speak to this nuance and this reciprocal relationship.

[143] Berne et al., "'Beauty Always Recognizes Itself,'" 246.

[144] Sins Invalid, *Skin, Tooth, and Bone*, 116.

[145] Garland-Thomson, Rosemarie, *Staring*, 19.

[146] Garland-Thomson, Rosemarie, *Staring*, 37.

[147] Garland-Thomson, Rosemarie, *Staring*, 84.

[148] Berne and Lewis et al., "'Beauty Always Recognizes Itself,'" 238.

149 hooks, *Teaching to Transgress*; Love, Bettina, *We Want to Do More than Survive: Abolitionist Teaching and Pursuit of Educational Freedom*.

150 Freire, *Pedagogy of the Oppressed*, 26.

151 Freire, Paulo, *Pedagogy of the Oppressed*, 30.

152 Freire, *Pedagogy of the Oppressed*, 70.

153 Freire, *Pedagogy of the Oppressed*, 62.

154 Although Paulo Freire does not directly state what love is in the *Pedagogy of the Oppressed* (2019), this chapter heavily relies on and imagines what education as a love practice looks like and does.

155 Love, *We Want to Do More than Survive*, 2.

156 On their website, Sins Invalid lists the following political education topics: ableism 101, Disability Justice, disability and sexuality, history of disability rights, history of eugenics and disability, history of disability oppression, fat liberation and Disability Justice, and Disability Justice for allies.

157 Freire, *Pedagogy of the Oppressed*, 30.

158 Freire, *Pedagogy of the Oppressed*, 65.

159 Freire, *Pedagogy of the Oppressed*, 64.

160 Freire, *Pedagogy of the Oppressed*, 30.

161 hooks, *Teaching to Transgress*, 12.

162 The Disability Justice Collective (DJC) is an inclusive space for disabled folks who are LGBTQIA+, who are of color, and who are low-income. The DJC provides these communities with resources to build connections, accessibility, and to gain leadership skills. For more information, visit littleglobe.org/portfolio/disability-justice-collective/.

163 hooks, *Teaching to Transgress*, 12.

164 Piepzna-Samarasinha, Leah Lakshmi, *Care Work: Dreaming Disability Justice*, 15.

165 Piepzna-Samarasinha, *Care Work*, 72.

166 In Alison Kafer's 2019 article "Crip Kin, Manifesting," she explores how "slavery, mass incarceration, settler colonialism, and eugenics" have severed kinship networks and systems. Indigenous, queer, and critical race theorists call these histories forward and reveal the importance and the prevalence of kinships outside of a settler colonial, white supremacist framework.

167 Rapp, Rayna and Faye Ginsburg, "Enabling Disability: Rewriting Kinship, Reimagining Citizenship."

168 Kafer, Allson, "Crip Kin, Manifesting," 6.

169 Sins Invalid, "Cultural and Political Programs Internships for Summer 2012."

170 The concept of messiness as generative comes from Angela McRobbie's work, particularly her writing about cultural studies.

171 Sins Invalid, *Skin, Tooth, and Bone*, 124.

172 Sins Invalid, "Fucking While Cripped Part 2."

173 Millett-Gallant, Ann, *The Disabled Body in Contemporary Art*.

174 Millett-Gallant, 11.

175 Sins Invalid, *Mark Your Calendar for Sins Invalid's Online Pay Per View*.

176 Boggs, Grace Lee, "Grace Lee Boggs: Introduction to Revolution and Evolution in the Twentieth Century."

177 Sins Invalid, *Va-Va-Voom!: A Crip Dance Party*.

178 Dworetzky, Joe, "Sins Invalid to Stream Performance."

179 Sins Invalid, "Fucking While Cripped Part 1."

180 The mainstream Disability Rights Movement did not actively advocate for a crip sexual culture. Before turning to sexual freedoms, the movement prioritized—and rightfully so in the beginning—civil and political access, including equal education, employment opportunities, and accessible transportation (Shakespeare, 2000, 106).

181 Mollow, Anna and Robert McRuer, *Sex and Disability*, 32.

[182] Sexual agency refers to a person's right to define their sexuality for their bodyminds, on their own terms. While much of this chapter and Sins Invalid's focus is on sexuality and eroticism, not all embodied folks are sexual. Some folks are, for example, asexual, a sexual orientation that is very much distinct from the oppressive process of desexualization.

[183] Shakespeare, Tom, "Researching Disabled Sexuality."

[184] UCLA School of Law Williams Institute (2019), williamsinstitute.law.ucla.edu/publications/conversion-therapy-and-lgbt-youth.

[185] brown, adrienne maree, *Pleasure Activism*, 9.

[186] brown, *Pleasure Activism*, 8.

[187] Mollow and McRuer, *Sex and Disability*, 1.

[188] Silverberg, Cory, "When It Comes to Sex, Are Your Sins Invalid?"

[189] brown, adrienne maree, *Pleasure Activism*, 11.

[190] *Sins Invalid: An Unshamed Claim to Beauty*.

[191] Sins Invalid, "Fucking While Cripped Part 2."

[192] Siebers, Tobin, *Disability Theory*, 136.

[193] Siebers, *Disability Theory*, 149.

[194] Sins Invalid, "Fucking While Cripped Part 2."

[195] hooks, bell, "Choosing the Margin as a Space of Radical Openness", 20.

[196] Nomy Lamm, "Wall of Fire" (2008, Oakland, Sins Invalid), performance.

[197] To acknowledge the lineage of activists in the Fat Liberation Movement, I intentionally use and capitalize the word Fat. Fat studies has taught us that Fat is not an insult; rather, it is a political, reappropriated term of empowerment.

[198] Lamm, Nomy, e-mail message, January 31, 2015.

[199] Lamm, Skype interview, April 4, 2014.

[200] Krip-Hop Nation brings awareness and community building to disabled hip-hop artists and musicians. Created by Leroy F. Moore Jr., it seeks to highlight the talents of musicians with disabilities while also unearthing this community's history. For more information, visit kriphopnation.com.

201 The following is an abbreviated list of disabled sex educators and activists who advocate for crip sex as an inherent right: Bethany Stevens, Eva Sweeney, Katherine McLaughlin, Julia Bascom, and Robin Wilson-Beattie among many, many others.

202 Sins Invalid, *Skin, Tooth, and Bone*, 116.

203 For more information on reproductive justice, visit the collective Sister Song: sistersong.net.

204 Sins Invalid, *Skin, Tooth, and Bone*, 116–117.

205 Sins Invalid, *Skin, Tooth, and Bone*, 121.

206 Berne, Patty, Jamal T. Lewis et al., "'Beauty Always Recognizes Itself': A Roundtable on Sins Invalid," 244.

207 Allen, D., "Liberating Beauty: A Conversation with Sins Invalid's Patty Berne."

208 Mingus, Mia, "Moving Toward the Ugly: A Politic Beyond Desirability."

209 Mingus, "Moving Toward the Ugly."

210 Mia Mingus historicizes her discussion of why we need to challenge normative beauty and desirability politics. She identifies the freak shows and sideshows of the nineteenth and twentieth centuries as moments when normative beauty was celebrated while the "ugly" was put on display and reinforced as unhuman and abject.

211 Sins Invalid, "Our Mission."

212 Berne, Patty and Jamal T. Lewis et al., "'Beauty Always Recognizes Itself': A Roundtable on Sins Invalid," 245.

213 Berne et al., "'Beauty Always Recognizes Itself,'" 247.

214 "Bringing It Black" (2016) was written by NEVE and Malcolm Shanks. It was performed by NEVE and Antoine Hunter, and it was voiced by Malcolm.

215 In her book *Feminism is for Everybody: Passionate Politics*, bell hooks (2000) writes about how feminism intervened in the sexist framework of beauty. I apply her argument—that we can use our activist movements (feminism in this case) to challenge and recreate the definitions of beauty—to the topic of crip beauty.

216 hooks, bell, *All About Love: New Visions*, 249.

217 Berne et al., "'Beauty Always Recognizes Itself,'" 241.

[218] Berne et al., "'Beauty Always Recognizes Itself,'" 242.

[219] This concept of resting to dream change comes from the work of Tricia Hersey, the creator of the Nap Ministry.

[220] Hamblin, James and Katherine Wells, "Listen: You Are Worthy of Sleep."

[221] Kroth, Maya, "It's a Right, Not a Privilege."

[222] Kroth, "It's a Right, Not a Privilege."

[223] Piepzna-Samarasinha, Leah Lakshmi, *Care Work*, 122.

[224] Edelman 2004; Halberstam 2005; Munoz 2009; Paur 2005.

[225] Kafer, Alison, *Feminist, Queer, Crip*, 28.

[226] Kafer, *Feminist, Queer, Crip*, 46.

[227] For Tricia Hersey, this exhaustion, specifically for Black folks, comes from capitalism; however, it is also rooted in the racialized sleep gap, "grind culture," and from the slavery narratives of laziness. Her work is pointing to the ways in which white supremacy and anti-Black racism inform rest, particularly for Black folks.

[228] Wong, Alice, "Labor, Care Work, & Disabled and Queer Femmes."

[229] Wong, "Labor, Care Work, & Disabled and Queer Femmes."

[230] Piepzna-Samarasinha, Leah Lakshmi, *Care Work*, 241.

[231] Piepzna-Samarasinha, *Care Work*, 241.

[232] *Decolonize the Future.*

[233] *Decolonize the Future.*

[234] *Decolonize the Future.*

[235] *Decolonize the Future.*

[236] Wong, Alice, *Disability Visibility: First-Person Stories from the Twenty-First Century*, 272.

[237] Berne, "Disability Justice—A Working Draft."

ACKNOWLEDGMENTS

Crip Kinship exists today because of love and trust, because of my desire to seek out and root with disabled, queer of color meaning-makers and artist-activists. I extend my stimmy, glittery crip joy and gratitude, first, to Sins Invalid's abundant, transformative community, particularly Patty Berne, Leroy F. Moore Jr., Nomy Lamm, Leah Lakshmi Piepzna-Samarasinha, and Maria Palacios. Thank you for your trust, for the many hours of interviews, for all of the video calls and email conversations. I am honored to know you and to learn from you.

I could not have arrived at this place of completion without the many dear friends and colleagues who wrote in community with me and provided feedback along the way: Kelan Koning, Adrienne Benally, Nayely Castrellón, Dora and Javier Gomez-Lopez, Jennette Ramirez, Pablo Alvarez, Shira Ingram, Rodney Hume-Dawson, Analena Hope Hassberg, and José Aguilar-Hernández. Thank you for joining me online and in person throughout these many years as I wrote and edited this offering. Endless gratitude as well to my writing group—Tamar Salibian, Beth Jones, Carlos Echeverria-Estrada, Myles Mikulic, and Jocelyn Storm—who shared space with me four days a week in the summer of 2020 as I concluded the manuscript. You have all grounded me and provided me with invaluable support. Thank you for guiding me through the labor of writing and all the anxiety, self-doubt, and ecstatic joy that comes with this process.

In remembering the roots of this work, I extend my gratitude to my undergraduate mentor, Leilani Hall, who introduced me to disability studies; to Kivi Neimi, who originally shared Sins Invalid with me; and to Tristan Scremin, the first person who taught me how to manifest disability pride.

To Eve Oishi, Jennifer Friedlander, Alex Juhasz, and Petra Kuppers: as members of my dissertation committee, you empowered me forward. Thank you for motivating me to reimagine this text and to insert my bodymind into the work; Alex, I am so grateful for your urging that I always "add pepper" to my writing, that I remember the productivity of messiness.

I have been able to thrive in academia and to challenge ableism and sanism's hold on my bodymind specifically because of my network of crip and Mad kin. I am indebted to this community and would especially like to thank Melanie Jones, Katherine M. Kinkopf, Sara M. Acevedo Espinal, Lydia X. Z. Brown, Alice Wong, Bethany Stevens, Vanessa Durand, Lilac Vylette Maldonado, Sarah Orem, and Krista Miranda. Thank you, dear ones, for your change-making and fierce crip solidarity, to all of my femme-tors of color who are ever-present forces of support and nourishment in my life. I extend joyous gratitude to Terri Gomez, my femme-tor at Cal Poly Pomona; thank you for emboldening my growth and confidence as an educator-scholar.

As much as Crip Kinship is for community, it is also for, and because of, my students at Cal Poly Pomona. I am grateful to call Cal Poly

Pomona and the Ethnic and Women's Studies department home. Thank you for creating loving, exploratory spaces of inquiry with me. I extend immense appreciation, in particular, to my research assistant Sophia Baroz, who helped me gather and organize my endnotes. I am so grateful to have worked in collaboration with you.

I gift this journey of words to my family. To my baba and mama—Bahram and Malakeh—and my siblings Sheva, Farima, and David, who encouraged me as I wrote, who listened, and who shared their excitement with me every step of the way.

To my best friend, Kelan: your friendship sustains me in profound and persistent ways. Thank you for journeying with me, for being my femme-tor, life doula, and sister in all things words. I could not have arrived in this distinct place, personally or academically, without your wisdom, tenderness, and guidance. Thank you for manifesting futurity for me, especially during the moments when I was not able to imagine my way forward.

And finally, and especially, to Amy: my love, I thank you for witnessing this process with such consideration, for nourishing my heart and spirit as I moved through this book journey, and for reminding me of the word "patience." Thank you for always holding expansive space, for grounding me, and for providing me with much-needed repair. Here's to the next journey, and the next.

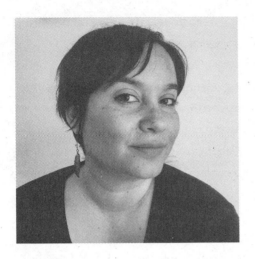

SHAYDA KAFAI (she/her) is an assistant professor of gender and sexuality studies in the Ethnic and Women's Studies department at California State Polytechnic University, Pomona. As a queer, disabled, Mad femme of color, she commits to practicing the many ways we can reclaim our bodyminds from systems of oppression. To support this work as an educator-scholar, Shayda applies disability justice and collective care practices in the spaces she cultivates. Shayda's writing and speaking presentations focus on intersectional body politics, particularly on how bodies are constructed and how they hold the capacity for rebellion. From discussions of madness and disability to femme politics and crip art, Shayda works to reframe our most disempowered bodyminds as vehicles of change-making. In honor of self-care and her communities, Shayda is also an artmaker and cofounder of CripFemmeCrafts with her wife, Amy. They make art that empowers all our bodyminds, particularly centering the magic and joy-making that comes from the wisdom and beauty of disabled, Fat bodyminds of color.